Coronary Angiography for the Interventionalist

George W. Vetrovec, MD
Director, Adult Cardiac Catheterization Laboratory
Medical College of Virginia Hospital
Professor of Medicine
Division of Cardiology
Department of Medicine
Medical College of Virginia
Richmond, Virginia

Evelyne Goudreau, MD
Interventional Cardiologist
Medical College of Virginia Hospital
Assistant Professor of Medicine
Division of Cardiology
Department of Medicine
Medical College of Virginia
Richmond, Virginia

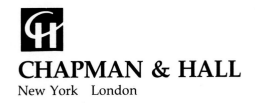

CHAPMAN & HALL
New York   London

First published in 1994 by

Chapman & Hall
One Penn Plaza
New York, NY 10119

Published in Great Britain by

Chapman & Hall
2–6 Boundary Row
London SE1 8HN

© 1994 Chapman & Hall, Inc.

Printed in the United States of America on acid-free paper.

Library of Congress Cataloging in Publication Data

Vetrovec, George W., 1943–
    Coronary angiography for the interventionalist / George W. Vetrovec, Evelyne Goudreau.
        p.   cm.
    Includes index.
    ISBN 0-412-04461-7 (alk. paper)
    1. Angiography.   2. Coronary heart disease—Interventional radiology.   3. Coronary arteries—Radiography.   I. Goudreau, Evelyne.   II. Title.
    [DNLM: 1. Angioplasty, Balloon, Laser-Assisted.   2. Angioplasty, Transluminal, Percutaneous Coronary.   3. Atherectomy, Coronary Angiography—methods.   4. Coronary Disease—therapy.   WG 300 V589c 1993]
RC683.5.A5V48   1993
617.4'12—dc20
DNLM/DLC   92-48409
for Library of Congress   CIP

To our families and friends who have supported us
throughout this endeavor

Preface

With the advent of angioplasty and its rapid evolution to the management of complex coronary disease, the importance of excellent angiographic definition has increased markedly. High-quality angiography enhances the safety, efficacy, and outcome of patient management. As experience with angioplasty has grown, the ability to predict its potential success based on lesion characteristics has increased. Thus, angiography plays an important role in patient selection. Furthermore, as newer nonballoon devices for percutaneous revascularization are developed, lesion morphology continues to grow as a major component of device selection.

This text highlights examples of tailoring views to optimize angiographic lesion detail in order to enhance decision making before, during, and after intervention, thus maximizing the safety and efficacy of interventional procedures. It is hoped that the examples and discussions that follow will reemphasize the importance of high-quality angiography. The goal is to provide a resource for the interventionalist that will aid in education and in patient management.

Coronary Angiography for the Interventionalist represents the contributions of many people. The discussions and questions posed by our colleagues and trainees over the years have spearheaded quite a few of the issues addressed in the text. In addition, the clinical procedures that we have performed have provided the concepts that we have attempted to translate.

Finally, we wish to acknowledge the dedication of Mrs. Joan Smith, Mrs. Shirley Jessup, and Mrs. Jeanie Toombs for their hard, diligent work and their technical help with the preparation of the manuscript. Special thanks go to Mr. Paul Greenwood for his photographic expertise.

George W. Vetrovec
Evelyne Goudreau

Contents

1

Introduction

Excellence in coronary angiography has taken on new significance in the era of coronary angioplasty and other recent interventions. Before such coronary interventions, angiography consisted of identifying either the presence or absence of coronary artery disease and, in patients with disease, assessing the severity of proximal stenoses and the quality of the distal vessels to determine the need and feasibility of bypass surgery.

However, with the advent of angioplasty, the need for excellence in angiography has increased. Assessment of pre- and postintervention lesion morphology, branch disease involvement, and location of moderate and even small branches, as well as the length and tortuosity of lesions, are all examples of the important angiographic information required in the era of interventional cardiology.

The purpose of this text is to focus on specific aspects of angiography relative to the needs of the interventionalist. Thus, the angiographic aspects of interventional procedures, such as specific views to enhance vessel separation, assessment of lesion morphology, and assessment of the interventional procedure outcome, will be presented. As a result, the beginning interventionalist will achieve a better understanding of the angiographic anatomy involved in angioplasty techniques and the experienced interventionalist will be provided with a useful review and a source of examples for training others.

Guiding Catheter-Enhanced Coronary Visualization

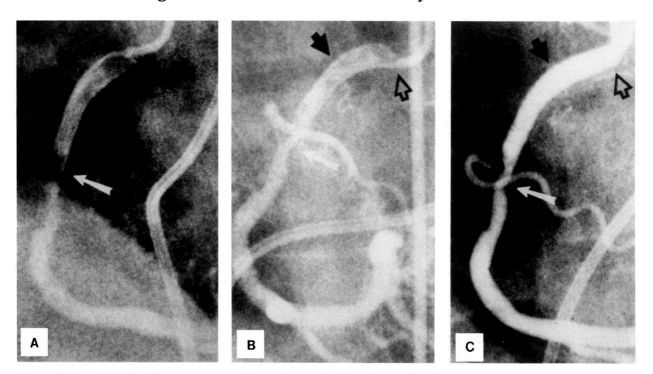

Figure 2-1.1   A 7 Fr high-flow catheter could not adequately fill the lumen of this large RCA. The hazy appearance (A), lacking dense contrast, suggests a large intracoronary thrombus in the proximal portion (black arrow) of the vessel. The severity of the lesion in the mid-portion (white arrow) is also not well delineated. A more forceful injection (B) could not improve coronary filling. Note that an ostial lesion of the RCA cannot be excluded. By changing to an 8 Fr guiding catheter to enhance contrast injection (C), adequate filling of the RCA is achieved; thus, an ostial lesion (open black arrow) or a filling defect in the proximal segment (closed black arrow) is excluded. The mid-lesion (white arrow) is now well demarcated.

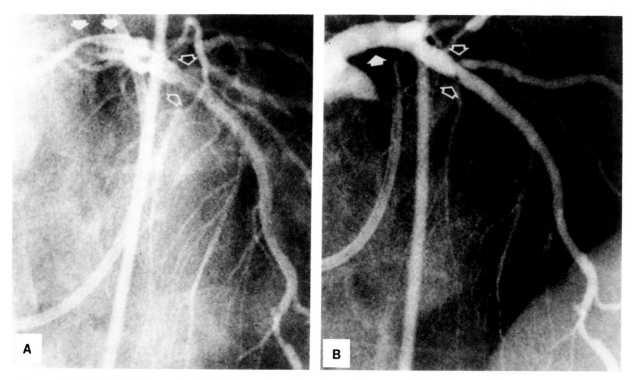

Figure 2-1.2   Injection through a 7 Fr diagnostic catheter is unable to provide adequate filling of the left coronary system (A), and there is an apparent intraluminal filling defect in the LMCA (closed arrows). In addition, the mid-portion of the LAD cannot be evaluated adequately (open arrows). Using an 8 Fr guiding catheter, the LMCA is adequately filled (B) and there is no evidence of an intraluminal filling defect (closed arrow). Also the mid-portion of the LAD is well delineated, showing an eccentric lesion with an associated high-grade ostial lesion of the diag branch (open arrows).

Postangioplasty Coronary Lesion Assessment

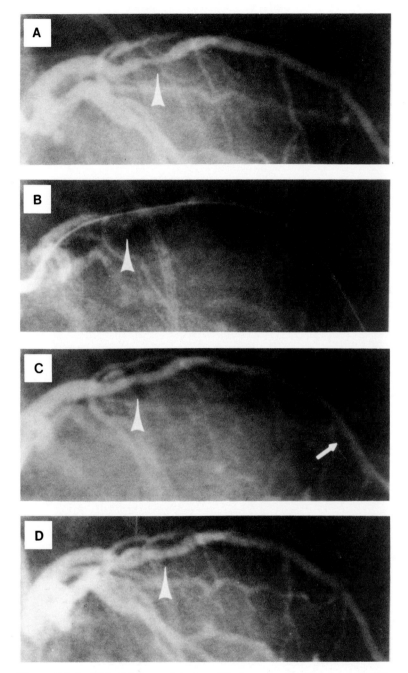

Figure 2-1.3 This RAO-cranial view (A) shows a significant mid-LAD lesion prior to PTCA. After balloon inflation, a test injection is performed with the balloon catheter pulled back into the guiding catheter (B). There is poor opacification of the LAD and, consequently, the results of angioplasty cannot be adequately assessed. To enhance visualization for better lesion assessment while maintaining guide wire access, a test injection is performed with the balloon catheter entirely withdrawn over an extension wire (C), while the guide wire (small arrow) is maintained across the lesion. There is now adequate opacification of the dilated site, confirming an excellent result. After the guide wire is withdrawn, a final angiogram (D) shows marked improvement of the dilated site with similar image quality to the previous test injection. This technique is particularly important with small Fr size guiding catheters, which reduce the available lumen for contrast injection around the balloon catheter.

Postangioplasty Lesion Assessment: Importance of Multiple Views

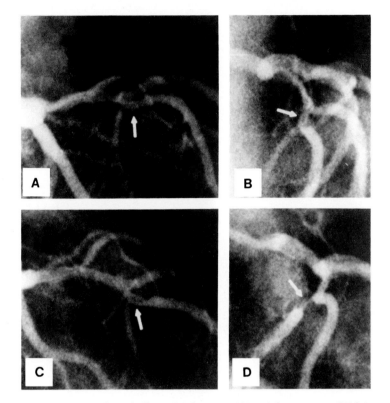

Figure 2-1.4 This shallow RAO view (A), 48 hours post-PTCA, demonstrates a small linear filling defect in the mid-portion of the LAD. In the AP-cranial view (B), the intraluminal filling defect is somewhat more obvious, but the lumen does not appear severely narrowed. In the RAO-cranial view (C), the linear dissection is better seen and there is evidence of a large filling defect. The LAO-cranial view (D) confirms the severe eccentricity of the dissection with evidence of a high-grade residual narrowing (arrow).

3

Native Coronary Angiography

To best assess lesions before and after an intervention, the involved segment must be targeted using appropriate views. The purpose of the next four sections is to summarize views that focus on specific vessel segments. While it is common to use angiographic systems that can be preprogrammed for specific operator-preferred views, it must be emphasized that each patient's heart is uniquely situated in the chest cavity. Because of the variations in coronary anatomy, a fixed set of angles for given views may not always be adequate to provide the desired detail or vessel separation. Thus, although suggested degrees of angulation are given, these often must be modified, depending on the X ray systems used and individual patient anatomy, to fine tune anatomic visualization.

It is assumed that each patient who undergoes coronary angiography will have a routine set of views performed for each vessel. Routine views frequently include a shallow RAO, an LAO-cranial, and steeper RAO views. Thus, the views emphasized in this text are not meant to be exclusive of other possible views, but only to highlight particular views that may be helpful in difficult anatomic assessment.

Each of the following sections summarizes routine and special views for major arterial segments, specifying the vessels and segments that are best highlighted by a particular view. In an effort to reduce radiation and total contrast administration, an angiographer need not utilize all of these views for every patient. However, after a limited series of routine views, additional projections can be selected to better outline details in segments of interest. In general, with greater vessel tortuosity and overlap, more views are required to assess all segments adequately.

3-1 LEFT MAIN CORONARY ARTERY

Prior to intervention, assessment of the LMCA is important in order to exclude significant disease that might preclude other interventional procedures, particularly in the setting of an unprotected, diseased, LMCA. Even prior to injection, an operator may suspect a significant LMCA lesion simply by monitoring arterial pressure. If there is any damping or ventricularization of the arterial pressure when the diagnostic catheter is engaged, one should be suspicious of possible obstruction and should perform initial limited dye testing only after careful attempts at repositioning the catheter to improve the pressure contour. It should be noted that if the size of the ostium of the LMCA is so small as to provide damping with a diagnostic catheter, the larger, nontapered tips of most guiding catheters are also likely to produce damping and flow obstruction. Although left coronary guiding catheters with side holes are available, the utilization of such catheters can be deceiving. For example, patients may become ischemic with prolonged catheter insertion in the LMCA because the side holes are not sufficient to provide adequate flow, despite maintenance of a normal pressure contour. Thus, a small or diseased ostial LMCA is an important factor in assessing the feasibility of interventions, especially for devices that require 9 or 10 Fr guiding catheters.

Ostial disease is best assessed by vigorous injection into the LMCA to provide reflux. The absence of reflux suggests ostial disease; however, the lack of reflux can be misleading when an injection is inadequate. A number of ostial LMCA projections are at times necessary to document significant disease. Table 3-1.1 and Figures 3-1.1 to 3-1.6 illustrate assessment of the LMCA.

Table 3-1.1 Coronary Angiographic Views: Left Main Coronary Artery

Vessel Segment	Routine Views	Adjunctive Views
Ostial	RAO (shallow)	AP-caudal
	LAO-cranial	RAO (steep)-cranial
	LAO-caudal	Lateral (110°)-caudal
		RAO-caudal
Body	RAO (shallow)	AP-caudal
	RAO-caudal	LAO (extreme)-caudal
	RAO-cranial	
	AP	
Distal	LAO-caudal	LAO (extreme)-caudal
	RAO-caudal	LAO-cranial
	LAO-cranial	AP-caudal

Ostial Left Main Assessment

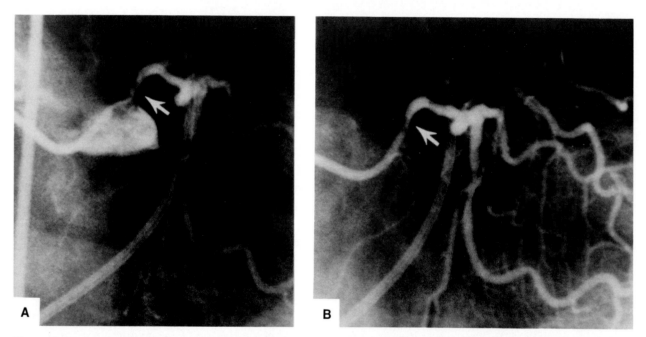

Figure 3-1.1   In this shallow RAO view (A), a nonselective injection in the left coronary cusp identifies a critical lesion at the ostium of the LMCA. The catheter is engaged (B) for injection and then withdrawn as soon as the injection is completed to avoid global ischemia. Note that there is no dye reflux when the catheter is engaged in the LMCA.

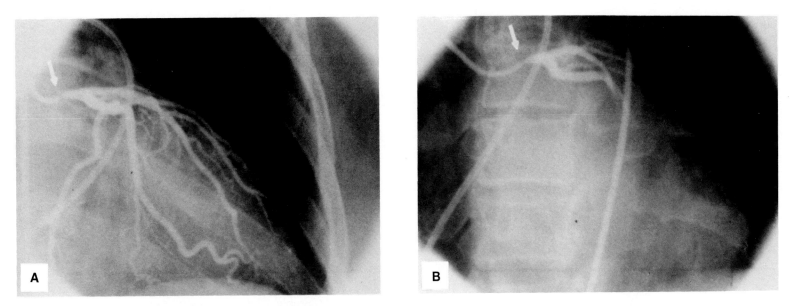

Figure 3-1.2   In the RAO view (A), the catheter is at the ostium of the LMCA but was not able to be selectively engaged because of the severity of the lesion. Note that in an LAO-caudal view (B), the length of the lesion is much better identified.

Distal Left Main Evaluation

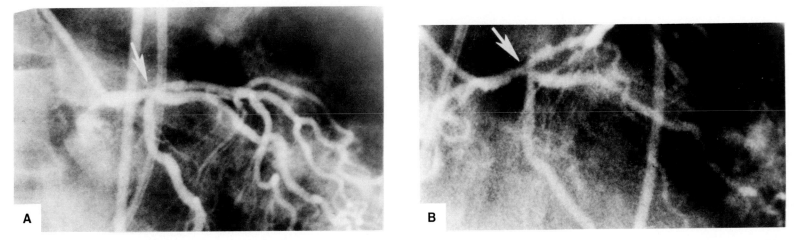

Figure 3-1.3   A shallow RAO view (A) shows a distal LMCA lesion, but assessment of the associated LAD and LCX involvement is limited by foreshortening and overlap. A subsequent shallow LAO, shallow caudal view (B) opens up the bifurcation, allowing better evaluation of the distal LMCA, LAD, and LCX bifurcation.

Distal Left Main Evaluation

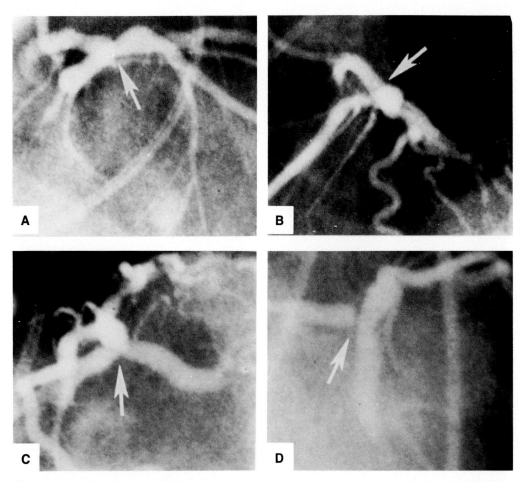

Figure 3-1.4 The RAO-caudal view (A) shows overlap of the origin of the LAD and LCX superimposed on the distal segment of the LMCA. In the LAO-cranial view (B), the distal LMCA is not visualized. In the LAO-caudal view (C), there is also overlap of the LAD and the distal LMCA. The AP-caudal view (D) demonstrates a critical stenosis of the LMCA. This view was helpful by eliminating LAD and LCX overlap over the distal LMCA.

Selective Cannulation of Common or Separate Left Anterior Descending and Circumflex Ostia

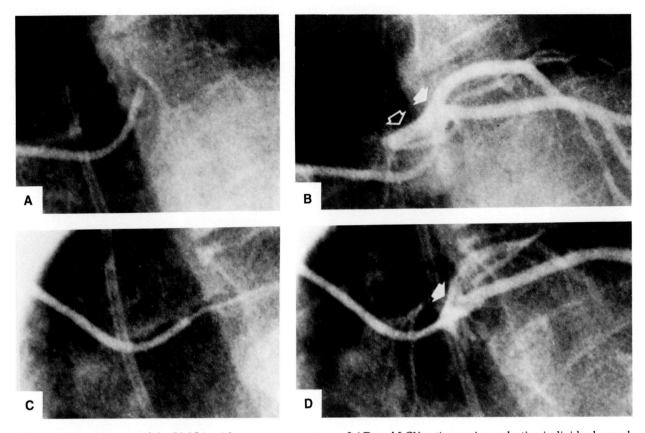

Figure 3-1.5   Absence of the LMCA with separate or common LAD and LCX ostia requires selective individual vessel cannulation. Shown here is the catheter position for selective LAD (A) and LCX (C) in an LAO-caudal view. Note that cannulation of the LAD is associated with a more upward catheter position, while the circumflex is cannulated with a more open catheter curve. Utilizing a longer curve catheter for the LCX (ie, a JL 5) or, conversely, a smaller catheter for the LAD (ie, a JL 3.5) can aid in selective cannulation. (B) and (D) represent selective injections of the LAD and the LCX through the catheters positioned as shown in (A) and (C). Note that it is sometimes possible, with a forceful injection, to adequately fill both vessels (B, closed arrow). There is also reflux in the left coronary cusp (open arrow).

Selective Cannulation of Common or Separate Left Anterior Descending and Circumflex Ostia

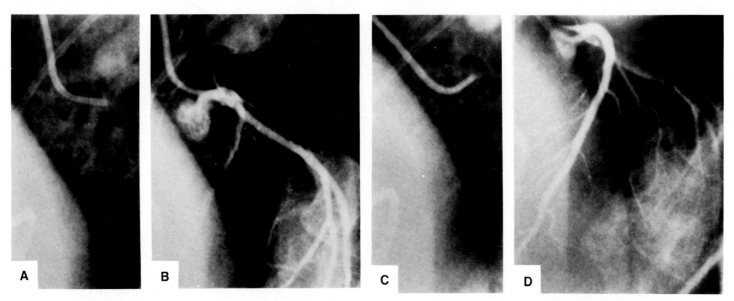

Figure 3-1.6   Selective LAD and LCX injections in the LAO-cranial projection, visualizing catheter positions for the LCX (A) and LAD (C) with associated injections seen respectively (B and D). Again, note the direction of the catheter position; an open catheter is used for the LCX and an upward-pointing catheter is used for the LAD. By careful selective cannulation of each artery, adequate opacification of each vessel is possible.

3-2 LEFT ANTERIOR DESCENDING ARTERY

The LAD artery and associated diagonals require multiple, carefully constructed views in order to adequately assess the LAD ostium at the takeoff from the LMCA, the proximal vessel segment, and the associated diagonals. The distal and apical segments of the LAD are usually well visualized in simple, shallow RAO and lateral views. In complex proximal and mid-LAD disease, assessment of the relationship of the lesions to the diag branches is crucial in determining the complexity and potential success of the angioplasty procedure.

To address these issues, Table 3-2.1 summarizes usual and special views of the LAD. Figures 3-2.1 to 3-2.10 illustrate these views.

Table 3-2.1   Coronary Angiographic Views: Left Anterior Descending Artery

Vessel Segment	Routine Views	Adjunctive Views
Ostial/proximal-diagonals	RAO (shallow) LAO-cranial RAO-cranial (steep) Lateral	AP-caudal Superlateral (LAO 110°) Lateral-cranial RAO-caudal LAO-caudal
Proximal/mid-diagonals	LAO-cranial RAO-cranial Lateral	LAO (shallow)-cranial (>30°) AP-cranial LAO (steep 75°–85°)-cranial RAO (shallow)-cranial (steep)
Distal/apical	RAO (shallow) Lateral	RAO-cranial LAO (shallow)-cranial AP-caudal RAO-caudal

Assessment of Ostial and Proximal Left Anterior Descending Artery

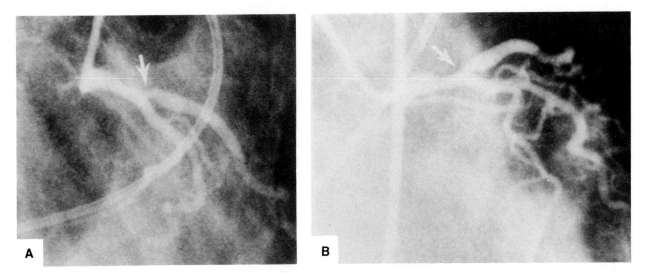

Figure 3-2.1   The RAO (30°)-caudal (30°) view (A) identifies a significant ostial lesion of the LAD. The AP-caudal (20°) view (B) is also useful for ostial or very proximal LAD lesions.

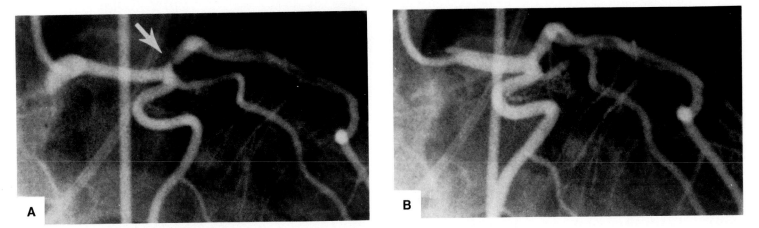

Figure 3-2.2   Shown here is an AP-caudal view demonstrating an ostial LAD stenosis (arrow), pre- (A) and postsuccessful (B) dilatation. The AP-caudal view is particularly useful for the distal LMCA and proximal LAD segment.

Evaluating the Proximal and Mid-Left Anterior Descending Artery

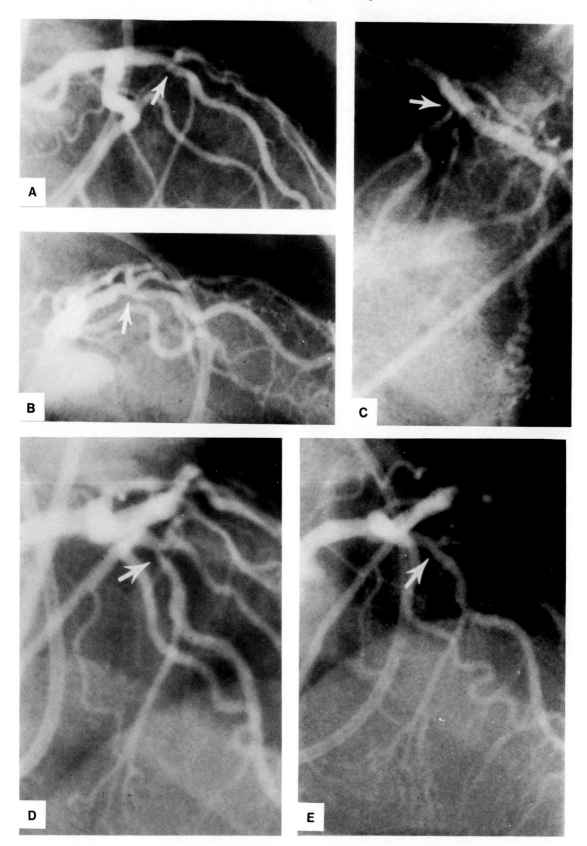

Figure 3-2.3 In this shallow RAO view (A), there is no significant narrowing observed in the proximal portion of the LAD. The RAO-cranial view (B) shows minimal, eccentric narrowing of the proximal portion of the LAD. The LAO-cranial view (C) is suspicious for a significant lesion in the proximal segment of the LAD, but there is overlap by the LCX precluding adequate assessment. The AP-cranial view (D) reveals a high-grade lesion in the LAD at the takeoff of a large diag. Following successful PTCA, the AP-cranial view (E) now shows minimal residual narrowing.

Optimizing Angulation of the AP-Cranial View

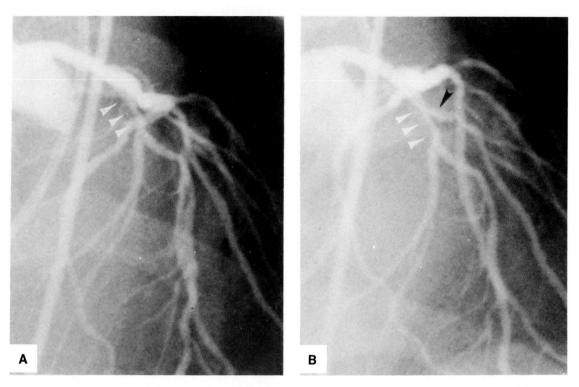

Figure 3-2.4 The AP-cranial (20°) view (A) reveals a significant tubular lesion in the proximal portion of the LAD prior to the takeoff of a first septal perforator, but the lesion is not well visualized due to LCX overlap. However, an AP view with steeper (30°) cranial angulation (B) better exposes the proximal LAD (white arrows), as well as the origin of a first diag (black arrow), which was not seen in (A).

LAO-Cranial Projection: Individualizing the Angulation

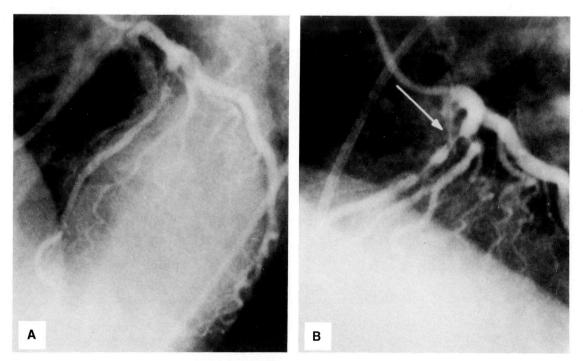

Figure 3-2.5 Routine LAO-cranial projections may require modifications depending on a patient's specific coronary anatomy. A standard LAO-cranial view (A) demonstrates an LAD stenosis beyond a diag with unquantified involvement of the diag. However, for appropriate preintervention assessment, better visualization of the lesion relative to morphology, length, and relation to the diag stenosis is important. (B) is a more cranial (40°) and steeper (75°) LAO view, which lengthens the LAD, while better identifying the diag ostial lesion. In addition, though not shown here, a shallow (20°–30°) LAO-cranial (30°–40°) projection also outlines the length and direction of the mid-diag takeoff.

LAO-Cranial Projection: Individualizing the Angulation

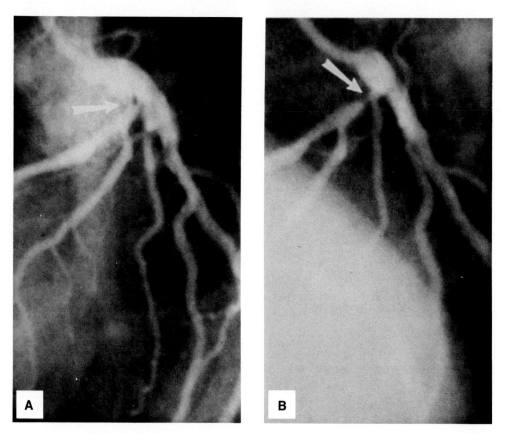

Figure 3-2.6 The standard LAO (45°)–cranial (30°) view (A) is suspicious for a critical proximal LAD lesion, but the lesion's relationship to the associated diag is not visualized. A steeper (60°) LAO-cranial (20°) view (B) demonstrates the takeoff of a large diag proximal to the LAD lesion.

Modification of the Lateral View: Preangioplasty

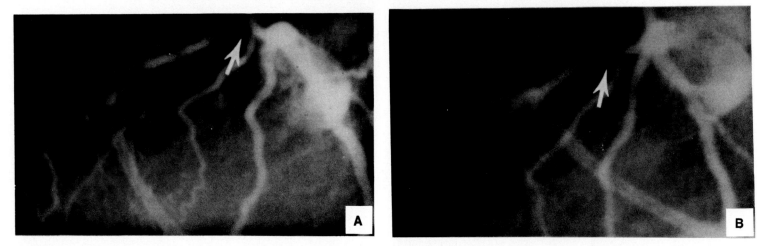

Figure 3-2.7 The length of the proximal LAD lesion is well appreciated in the lateral (90°) view (A), but the takeoff of the first diag is not seen. By utilizing a superlateral (100°), cranial (20°) angulation (B), the first diag branch and the proximal LAD lesion are better visualized.

Modification of the Lateral View: Postangioplasty Assessment

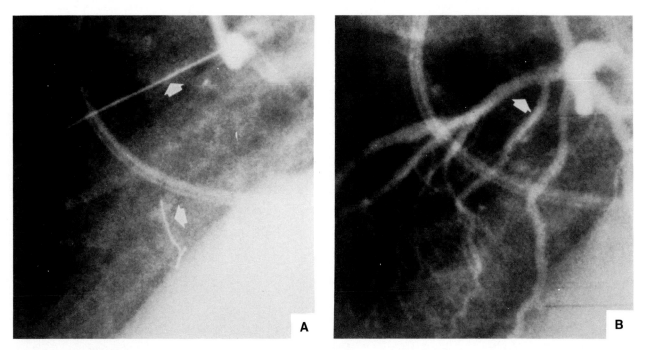

Figure 3-2.8   Steep LAO-cranial views [as in Figure 3-2.7 (B)] show dual wire access of the LAD and diag vessels (A). The excellent post-PTCA result is very apparent in this optimized view of the proximal LAD segment (B).

Steep LAO-Cranial Views for Proximal Diagonal Branches

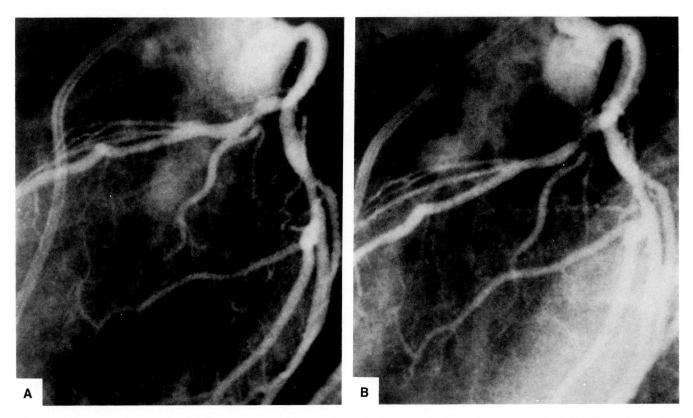

Figure 3-2.9   Assessment of ostial diag stenoses often requires tailoring a projection to best assess the LAD-diag relationship and any bifurcation disease. Shown here is a lateral projection (A), revealing the LAD stenosis but poorly visualizing the diag ostial involvement, which was not well demonstrated in multiple other views. When LAO angulation was reduced to 80° and cranial (20°) angulation is added, the LAD-diag stenoses are better visualized (B).

LAO-Cranial View For Mid-Diagonal Branches

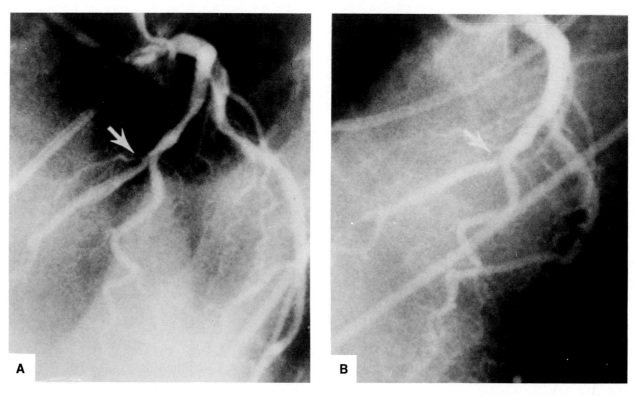

Figure 3-2.10   In this standard LAO (45°)–cranial (30°) view, the diag takeoff from the mid-LAD is partially obscured by overlap with the LAD (A). A more shallow LAO (20°) and steeper cranial (45°) view (B) better delineates bifurcation of the diag and the mid-LAD.

3-3 LEFT CIRCUMFLEX ARTERY

The ostial and proximal LCX segments, as well as proximal lesions in the RAMUS, can usually be adequately visualized in the LAO- and RAO-caudal views. Most often, the mid-LCX is easily assessed in shallow LAO, RAO, or even AP views. Distal vessel assessment depends on size and dominance. In small, nondominant LCX vessels, simple RAO and LAO views are sufficiently supplemented by RAO and AP-caudal projections. Conversely, in dominant vessels, views similar to those used to assess the distal RCA and PDA/PLB bifurcation are warranted. Special LCX views include shallow LAO-cranial and LAO-caudal views, as well as shallow RAO-cranial and AP-cranial views. Because of the marked variability of the LCX in size and distribution, views must be individualized. Suggested helpful views are given in Table 3-3.1 and Figures 3-3.1 to 3-3.7.

Table 3-3.1 Coronary Angiographic Views: Left Circumflex Artery

Vessel Segment	Routine Views	Adjunctive Views
Ostial/proximal	LAO	LAO-caudal (extreme)
	LAO-cranial	LAO (shallow)
	RAO-caudal	AP-caudal
Ostial RAMUS (intermediate)	LAO-caudal	LAO-caudal (extreme)
	LAO	LAO (90°–110°)-caudal (steep)
	RAO-caudal	AP-caudal
		RAO-cranial (steep)
Mid/marginals	RAO (shallow)	AP
	RAO-caudal	AP-caudal
	LAO (45°–60°)	LAO (10°–30°)
	LAO-caudal	
Distal (dominant)	RAO (shallow)	AP-cranial
	LAO (shallow) cranial	RAO-cranial
	RAO-caudal	Lateral-cranial

Ostial Circumflex Assessment

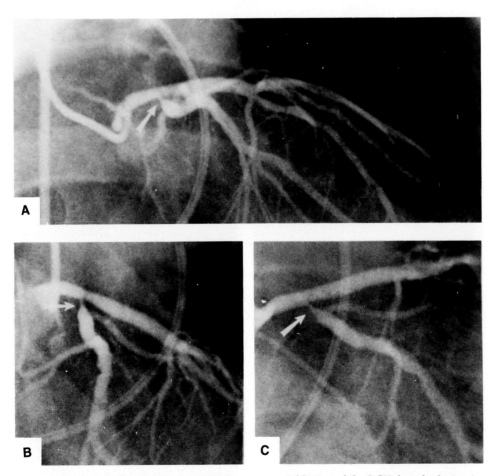

Figure 3-3.1 A shallow RAO view (A) shows an ostial lesion of the LCX, but the lesion is not well delineated secondary to foreshortening. An RAO-caudal view (B) better outlines the takeoff of the LCX, but the lesion is still somewhat foreshortened. The AP-caudal view (C) most clearly identifies the length and extent of the lesion.

Optimizing Views for the Ostial Intermediate Artery

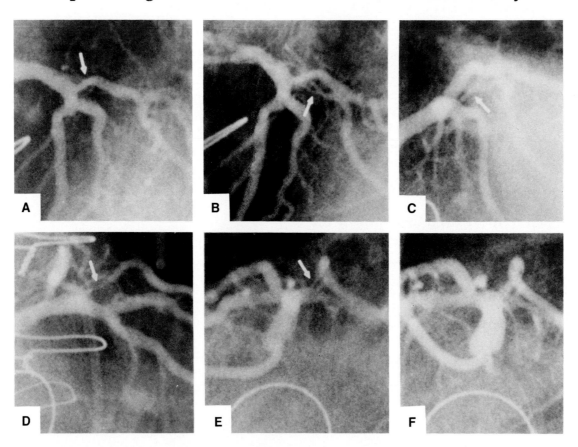

Figure 3-3.2   Routine views, such as shallow RAO and LAO-cranial (A), show no evidence of an intermediate branch. By tailoring different views, a high-grade lesion of a large intermediate branch is able to be identified. A steeper LAO-cranial view (B) identifies the intermediate branch, but its ostium is not well visualized. An LAO-caudal (extreme) view (C) shows the origin and length of the ostial lesion. Other special views include the AP view with steep cranial angulation (D) and a superlateral (110°) with caudal angulation (E). Identifying the views that best show the lesion, enhances the feasibility and success of PTCA and is crucial in evaluating the post-PTCA results (F).

Shallow RAO-Caudal View for Proximal Circumflex Artery

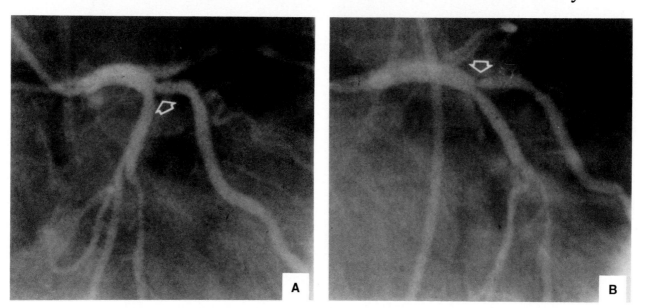

Figure 3-3.3   In the shallow RAO view (A), the takeoff of a high, first marg is foreshortened making the degree of stenosis difficult to assess. However, the shallow RAO-caudal view (B) clearly delineates the moderately severe stenosis at the ostium of the first marg.

Mid-Circumflex Evaluation

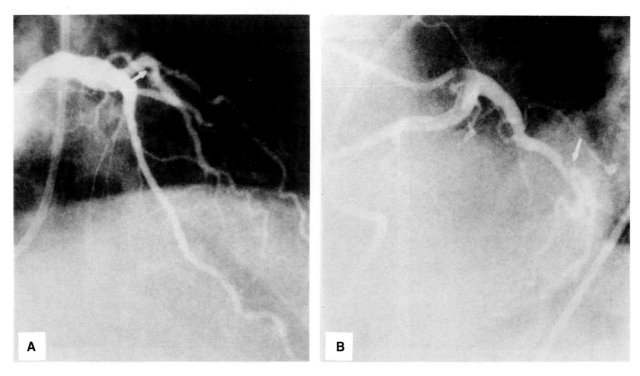

Figure 3-3.4   The mid-LCX and marg takeoffs are not well delineated in the shallow RAO view (A) or the LAO-cranial view (B) secondary to vessel overlap.

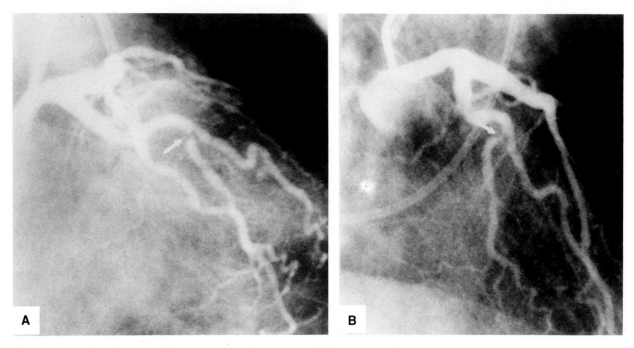

Figure 3-3.5   The AP-caudal (A) and shallow RAO-caudal (B) views clearly delineate a significant lesion in the marg bifurcating branch (arrow).

Ostial Right Coronary Artery Assessment

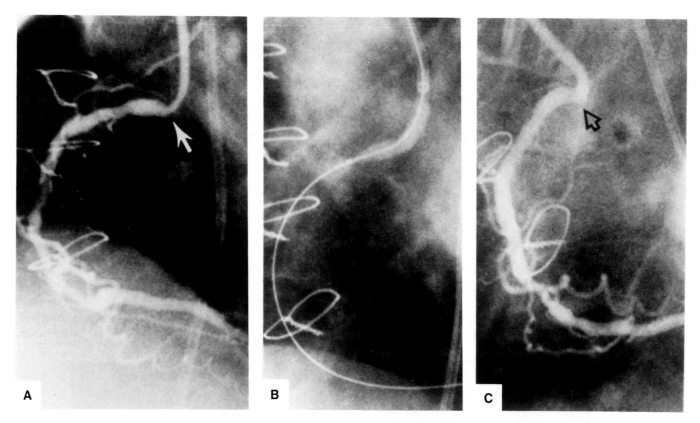

A   B   C

Figure 3-4.2   Shallow LAO view (A) again demonstrates a severe ostial RCA stenosis. (B) shows the balloon positioned across the stenosis with the maximum area of balloon diameter in the ostium. The guiding catheter is removed to allow effective balloon positioning and inflation. Finally, the result is well visualized in an LAO-caudal view (C).

Ostial Right Coronary Artery Assessment

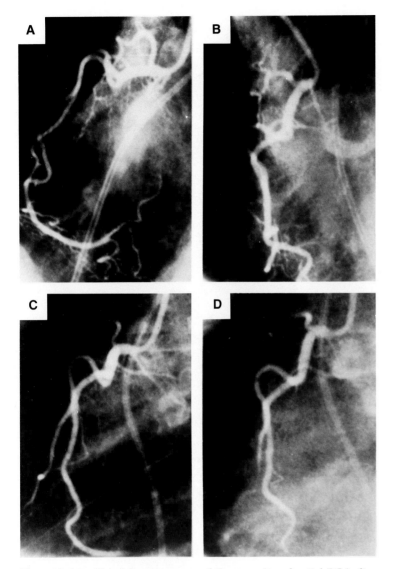

Figure 3-4.3 Careful assessment of the severity of ostial RCA disease suspected on preliminary RCA injections associated with mild catheter-induced pressure damping is important. (A) is a shallow LAO-cranial view in which the severity of the ostial stenosis is difficult to assess. (B) is an LAO-caudal view, which suggests possible obstruction by reduced contrast reflux. (C) is a lateral view, which illustrates moderate reflux with a linear jet, suggesting an ostial lesion. Finally, (D) shows that the length of the lesion is best assessed in the superlateral view.

Evaluation of the Proximal Right Coronary Artery

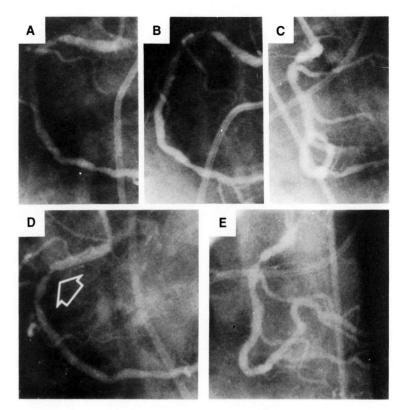

Figure 3-4.4 This series of RCA injections compares the relative effectiveness of each view in identifying the morphology and, particularly, the total length of a proximal RCA stenosis in a tortuous, proximal RCA. Note that a standard LAO view (A) identifies the lesion but is less ideal because of the extreme density mismatch between the lung and diaphragm backgrounds. Similar limitations are seen in the LAO-cranial view (B). (C) illustrates an RAO view, which significantly foreshortens the proximal stenosis. An LAO-caudal view (D) and an AP-cranial view (E) provide the best overall straightening of the proximal portion of the RCA, as well as the relatively homogenous background density, to assess the lesion morphology and length.

Mid-Right Coronary Artery and Right Ventricular Branch Assessment

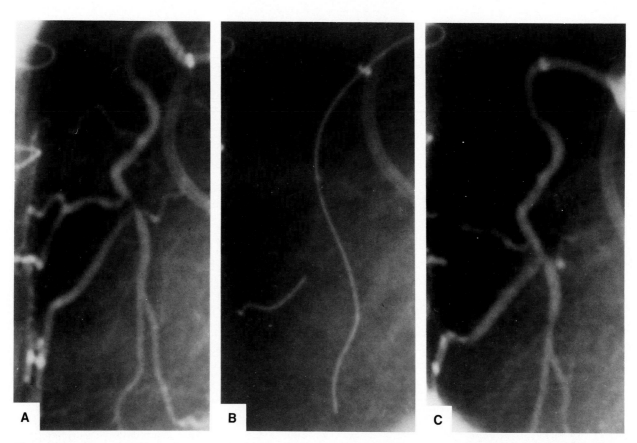

Figure 3-4.5   Sequential lateral projections showing a small RV branch stenosis along with a severe mid-stenosis of a small RCA (A). The lateral view provides excellent visualization of the primary lesion for guide wire passage as well as for successful placement of a non–over-the-wire balloon catheter in the largest of the two RV branches (B). (C) illustrates the follow-up result; again the lateral view best visualizes the primary RCA lesion area and the RV branch result after PTCA.

Optimizing Views for the Distal Right Coronary Artery

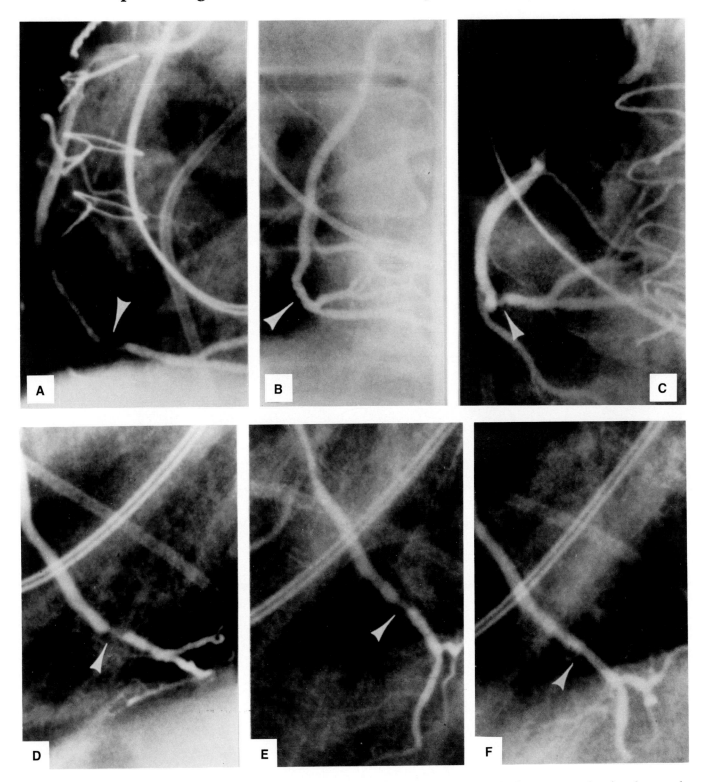

Figure 3-4.6   In this LAO (30°) view (A), the lesion is seen in the distal portion of the RCA but is somewhat foreshortened. Foreshortening is even worse in the shallow RAO view (B), completely obscuring the lesion. In the AP-cranial view (C), the lesion in the distal portion of the RCA is only partially delineated. In the lateral view (D), the distal portion of the RCA and the lesion are well visualized (arrow). A superlateral view (E) with cranial angulation also clearly identifies the length and severity of the lesion. Finally, after successful PTCA (F), there is minimal residual narrowing seen in a similar superlateral view with cranial angulation.

Distal Right Coronary Artery: Focusing on the Bifurcation

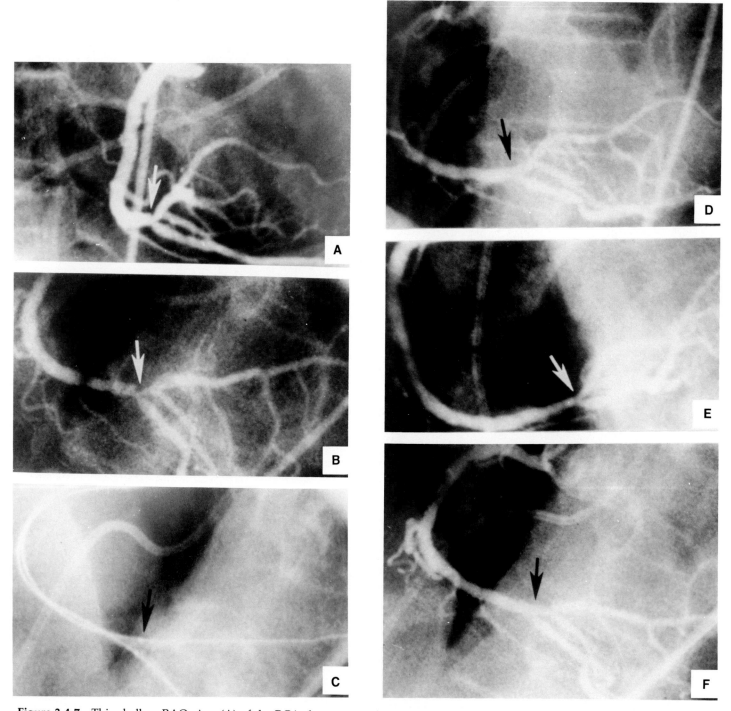

Figure 3-4.7   This shallow RAO view (A) of the RCA shows a significant lesion involving the PDA/PLB bifurcation. The LAO-cranial view (B) reveals eccentricity of the same lesion. Simultaneous balloon inflation across the bifurcating vessels is seen in an LAO-cranial view (C). On test injection following balloon inflation, there is marked improvement at the dilated site with minimal residual narrowing. The post-PTCA bifurcating segment is assessed in the LAO view (D), the LAO-caudal view (E), and the LAO-cranial view (F) with excellent results seen in all views. (Reprinted by permission from George Vetrovec, MD. Chapter 15. In Carl J. Pepine, MD, et al. *Diagnostic and Therapeutic Cardiac Catheterization.* 1989. Copyright © 1989, the Williams & Wilkins Co., Baltimore.)

4

Bypass Grafts

4-1 SAPHENOUS VEIN GRAFTS

Vein graft anatomy requires individualization because the ostial position of the graft is determined by the surgical insertion site, while the course and tortuosity of the vein graft body is determined by the length and direction of the graft. Various views are sometimes required to straighten or most ideally assess any questionable segment of the graft. A major goal is to assess the eccentricity of the graft lesions.

The second important requirement is to adequately assess the distal insertion site. This requires tailoring a view in order to have the best visualization at the insertion site in a perpendicular plane to the native vessel. Finally, adequate contrast injection of the graft is important to avoid streaming, which may suggest a thrombus or a lesion, and to provide adequate visualization of the distal native vessel. Simply reaching the graft with a catheter is often not adequate, but manipulation of the catheter for ideal cannulation allows adequate opacification. When the

graft is large, utilization of a guiding catheter may be necessary to provide maximum contrast injection and, thus, adequate opacification even during diagnostic studies. Again, streaming of contrast is associated with over- or underestimation of the graft or vessel disease. Conversely, adequate opacification demonstrating diffuse graft body disease is important since this suggests friable material which may increase the risk of embolization during intervention and may be an important factor in excluding a vein graft from intervention.

Ostial lesions are assessed not only by pressure damping with catheter engagement but also by rotating the catheter to provide a parallel catheter/ostial graft view. Such views must be individualized based on the relationship of the graft to the aorta. Table 4-1.1 describes usual views particularly related to the distal insertion site and emphasizes that the best views are often those that are more specific for the native artery. Views of the grafts themselves frequently have to be more individualized as Figures 4-1.1 to 4-1.13 suggest.

Table 4-1.1 Coronary Angiographic Views: Bypass Grafts

Vessel Segment		Views	Adjunctive Views
OSTIA	Left	RAO (shallow)	AP
		LAO	
	Right	LAO	Lateral
		RAO	
		LAO-cranial	
BODY		LAO	(individualize
		RAO	to assess
			tortuous
			and eccen-
			tric seg-
			ments)
DISTAL INSERTION TO:			
LAD/diag		RAO	AP-cranial
		LAO-cranial	Lateral
		RAO-cranial	
LCX/marg		RAO	AP-caudal
		LAO	(shallow)
		RAO-caudal	LAO-caudal
RCA		LAO	LAO-caudal
		RAO	Lateral
		LAO-cranial	AP-cranial
PDA/PLB (bifurcation)		RAO	AP-cranial
		LAO-cranial	Lateral
			Lateral-cranial
			LAO-caudal
PDA/PLB mid-vessel		RAO	RAO-cranial
		LAO-cranial	AP-cranial
			Lateral-cranial
			RAO-caudal
			AP-caudal

Ostial Right Vein Graft Stenosis

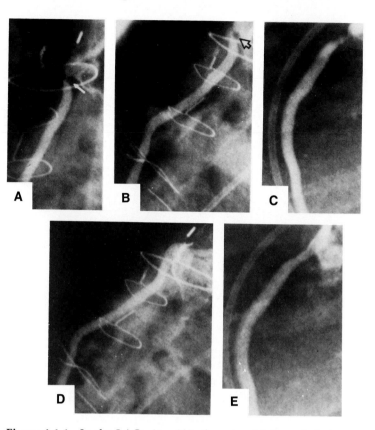

Figure 4-1.1 In the LAO view (A), there is a high-grade lesion at the ostium of this RCA saphenous vein graft. The lesion is also seen in this LAO-cranial view (B), as well as in the lateral view (C), which best identifies the total length of the lesion. The post-PTCA result is seen in the LAO-cranial view (D), which reveals a minimal residual narrowing. In addition, the lateral view shows some mild residual narrowing (E).

Ostial Right Vein Graft Stenosis

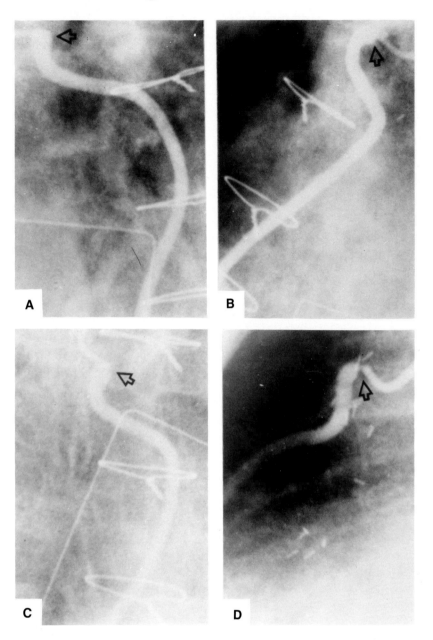

Figure 4-1.2   The shallow RAO (A) and the shallow LAO (C) views show no evidence of an ostial RCA graft. However, the LAO-cranial view (B) suggests an ostial stenosis that was severe as confirmed in the lateral view (D).

Right Vein Graft Body Disease

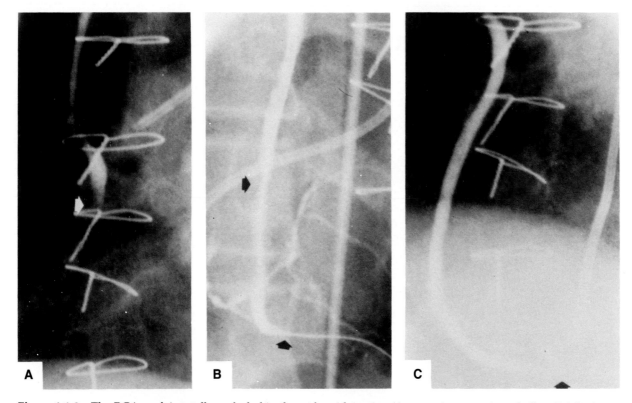

Figure 4-1.3   The RCA graft is totally occluded in the early mid-portion (A, arrow) as seen in a shallow LAO view. A shallow RAO view (B) shows a high-grade residual graft lesion after UK and PTCA (upper black arrow). There was also distal embolization as indicated by the lower black arrow. After additional UK infusion and balloon inflation, there was successful reperfusion of the vein graft and restoration of antegrade flow in the distal RCA (C).

(Reprinted from A. Arthur Halle, III, et al. Angioplasty of a recently occluded coronary artery bypass graft. *Catheterization and Cardiovascular Diagnosis* 21:180–184, 1990. Copyright © 1990 by *Catheterization and Cardiovascular Diagnosis.* Reprinted by permission of Wiley-Liss, a division of John Wiley and Sons, Inc.)

Right Vein Graft: Distal Insertion Site

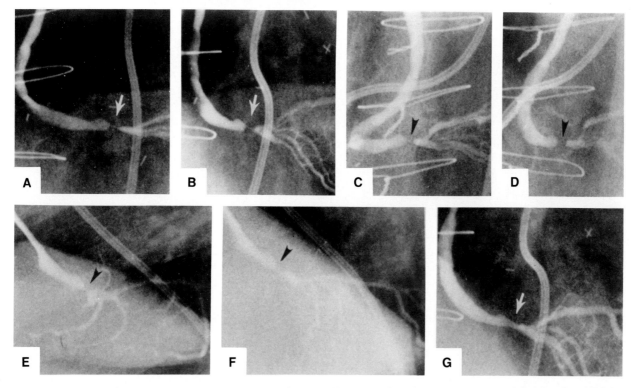

Figure 4-1.4   The distal insertion of a RCA vein graft is usually assessed in the same views used for the distal RCA. This shallow LAO view (A) shows a significant lesion at the distal insertion site. The relation of the lesion to the PDA/ PLB bifurcation is better assessed in the LAO-cranial (B) and the AP-cranial (C) views. The shallow RAO (D), lateral (E), and lateral-cranial (F) views are also useful in assessing the distal graft insertion to the native RCA. Post-PTCA (G), the LAO-cranial view demonstrates marked improvement.

Analyzing Vein Graft Filling Defects

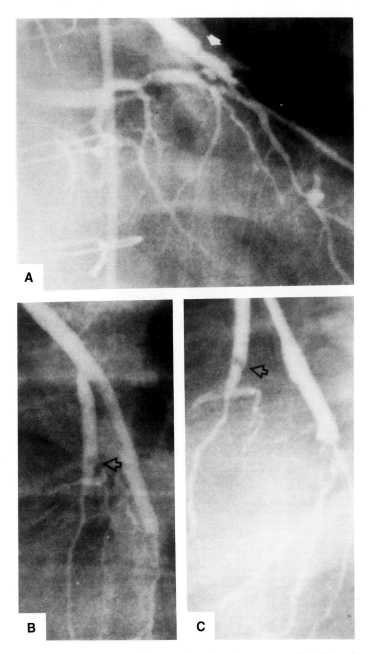

Figure 4-1.5 In the RAO view (A), there is an eccentric lesion of the vein graft proximal to LAD anastomosis site. The filling defect in the LAD vein graft limb is better defined in the AP-cranial (B) and LAO-cranial (C) views. The eccentric but flap-like nature is suggestive of a thrombotic filling defect associated with atherosclerotic disease, and is important to recognize because of the risk of distal embolization during PTCA. The following Figure 4-1.6 shows the same patient.

Views of Native Coronary Arteries Distal to Vein Graft Insertion

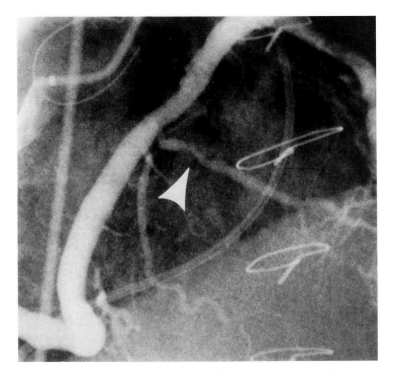

Figure 4-1.6 Assessing lesions in native arteries beyond graft insertion sites usually requires utilizing views for the appropriate native segments, modified when necessary to avoid graft overlap. For instance, in this shallow RAO view, a single graft sequentially anastomosed to a PDA segment (branch at bottom of photo)—a mid-marginal with a lesion in the superior branch (arrow)—and terminated in the LAD. Of note is the size of the vein graft and its extensive tributaries, which required the use of a guiding catheter to adequately opacify the graft and its native segments.

Views of Native Coronary Arteries Distal to Vein Graft Insertion

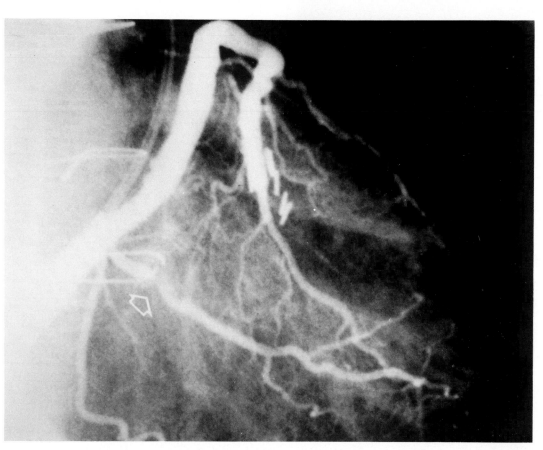

Figure 4-1.7 A later phase, shallow RAO frame illustrates the LCX marg stenosis (arrow), a superior diag insertion not seen in the preceding view, and the vein graft insertion in the native mid-LAD. The following Figure 4-1.8 shows the same patient.

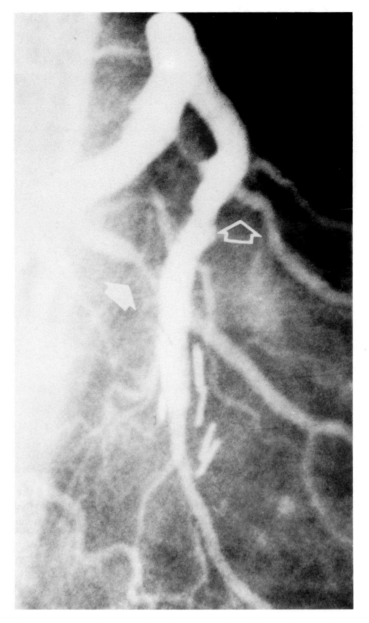

Figure 4-1.8   Shown is the AP-cranial view, illustrating excellent visualization of mid-LAD structures, to include the mid-diag insertion site (open arrow), the mid-LAD insertion site, and the marg stenosis (closed arrow) visible between turns in the graft. The following Figure 4-1.9 shows the same patient.

4-2 INTERNAL MAMMARY GRAFTS

With the increased use of the IMA as a conduit for coronary artery bypass surgery, more interventions are being required for this vessel. While the IMA itself is relatively rarely diseased, insertion site stenosis, particularly early after surgery, is a more common problem. Thus, an important aspect of IMA angiography is very careful assessment of the distal insertion site. Often visualization of IMA insertion to the mid-LAD is different than for vein graft. To that extent, the LAO-cranial view is less useful because of frequent overlap of the IMA and the LAD. Shallow and steeper RAO-cranial and lateral views are frequently more helpful for the distal insertion site.

In addition, spasm of the IMA graft may occur during the procedure; therefore, assessment of the IMA conduit for spasm is important during PTCA. In the presence of any significant change in luminal diameter, nitroglycerin should be used liberally to diagnose and treat spasm.

Finally, significant disease involving the proximal ipsilateral subclavian artery is a potential source of myocardial ischemia associated with an IMA graft. If, on entry into the subclavian artery, there is a decrease in arterial pressure compared to the central aortic pressure, angiography of the subclavian artery should be undertaken to assess any stenosis that could impair IMA flow.

Table 4-2.1 outlines associated views for assessment of the IMA. Chapter 9-2 reviews subclavian angiography.

Table 4-2.1 Coronary Angiographic Views: Internal Mammary Artery Graft

Vessel Segment	Routine Views	Adjunctive Views
INTERNAL MAMMARY		
Ostium	Shallow RAO	
	LAO	
Body	RAO	
	LAO (distal IMA)	Lateral
Insertion site to:		
LAD	LAO	RAO (steep)-cranial
	RAO	AP-cranial
	RAO-cranial	Lateral
		Superlateral (110°)
RCA	LAO	Lateral
	RAO	Lateral-caudal
	LAO-cranial	Superlateral-caudal
LEFT SUBCLAVIAN	AP	LAO-caudal
	LAO	RAO (steep)-cranial
	LAO-cranial	

Nonselective Internal Mammary Artery Injection

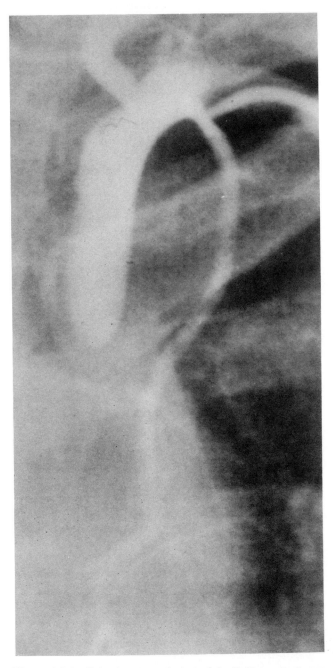

Figure 4-2.1 Selective cannulation of the IMA can at times be difficult. Visualization can be enhanced by using a blood pressure cuff inflated to systemic arterial pressure on the appropriate arm to limit run-off. Thus, the flow into the IMA is enhanced when nonselective injection is unavoidable. In addition, better access and guiding catheter support can be achieved by percutaneous ipsilateral arm catheterization. Shown here is a nonselective injection of the LIMA from left arm percutaneous access—utilizing cuff left arm compression to enhance filling.

Selective Internal Mammary Artery Access

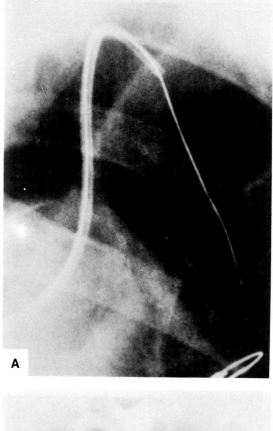

A

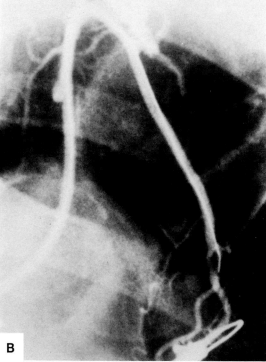

B

Figure 4-2.2 Selective IMA access may be difficult because of subclavian tortuosity or aberrant position of the IMA ostium. Nonselective injection in the subclavian artery may not sufficiently opacify the insertion site or distal native artery. Demonstrated here is use of a PTCA guide wire steered into the proximal IMA through a diagnostic catheter (A) to maintain selective access during injections (B) thus providing excellent opacification of the vessel.

Left Internal Mammary Graft Distal Insertion Site

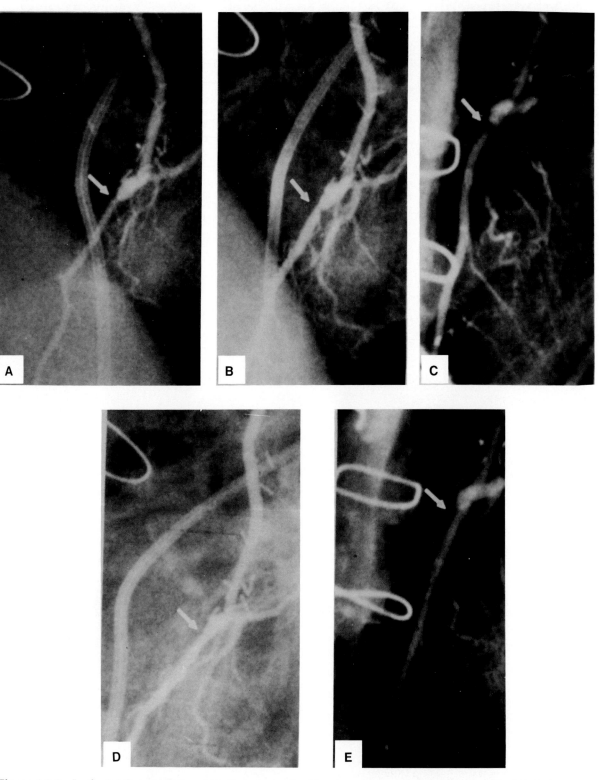

Figure 4-2.3   In the LAO-cranial view (A), there is no significant narrowing identified at the distal IMA insertion site but the LAD does appear small, suggesting possible vasoconstriction. This is confirmed in a similar LAO-cranial view (B) after the administration of intracoronary nitroglycerin, which identifies a significant lesion at the distal insertion site of the LIMA. This lesion is recognized after dilatation of the normal vessel segment by nitroglycerin. The lateral projection (C) also shows a high-grade eccentric lesion of the distal insertion site. Following successful coronary angioplasty, the LAO-cranial (D) and lateral (E) views demonstrate no significant residual narrowing at the distal insertion site.

Angioplasty-Associated Spasm

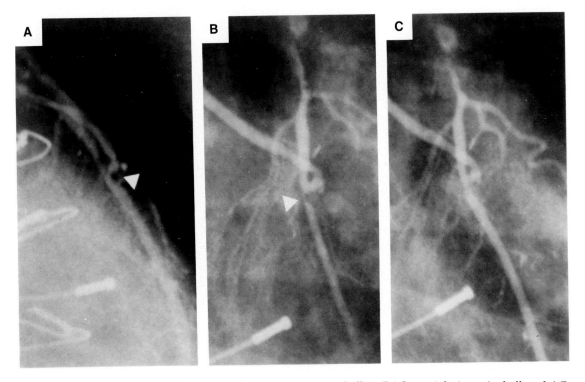

Figure 4-2.4 (A) represents the IMA stenosis (arrow) in a shallow RAO-cranial view. A shallow LAO-cranial view (B) illustrates the excellent graft insertion site result immediately following PTCA but identifies a new, eccentric LAD lesion just distal to the graft insertion site. Following nitroglycerin, in a similar view (C), there is resolution of this defect, as well as a continued excellent result at the IMA-PTCA site. Performing several views following PTCA is important, not only to assess the lesion segment result, but also to assess the remainder of the vessel for possible thrombus, spasm, or adjacent dissection, particularly in the patient who has ongoing symptoms despite an apparent satisfactory primary PTCA result.

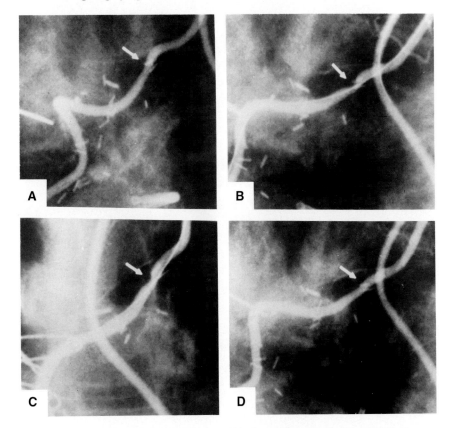

Figure 4-2.5 In this LAO-cranial view (A), the mid-portion of the LIMA shows no focal stenosis (arrow). After angioplasty of the distal insertion site, test injection in the same view shows an eccentric narrowing of the LIMA (B, arrow). The AP projection (C) also shows an eccentric, discrete narrowing of the LIMA. Following intracoronary nitroglycerin and low pressure balloon inflation, a similar LAO-cranial view (D) shows resolution of the focal spasm.

Angioplasty-Associated Thrombus

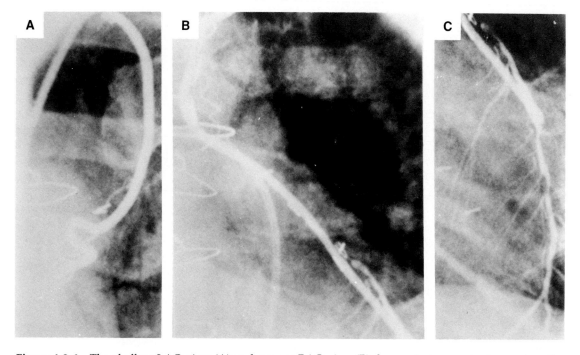

Figure 4-2.6 The shallow LAO view (A) and steeper RAO view (B) demonstrates a patent, nonstenotic proximal and mid-LIMA. (B) An AP-cranial view (C) shows significant native LAD disease beyond the graft insertion.

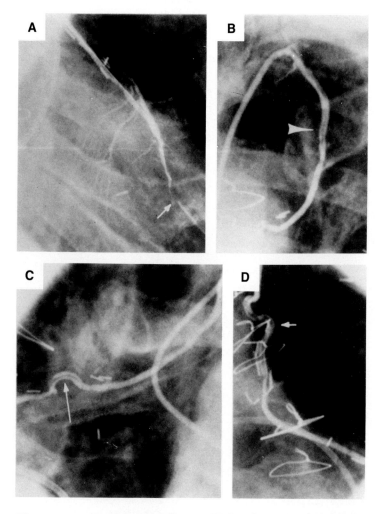

Figure 4-2.7 Immediately following PTCA, there was sluggish distal flow with a filling defect in the LAD (arrow) evident in an RAO-cranial view (A). In addition, there was evidence of a linear filling defect in the body of the IMA graft. Consistent with thrombus (arrows) as seen in the shallow RAO (B) and lateral (C) projections. The AP-cranial view (D) clearly identifies thrombus in the LIMA.

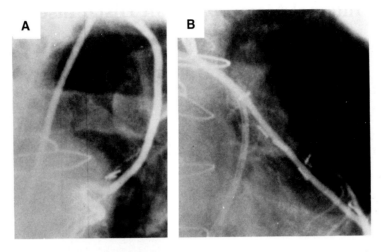

Figure 4-2.8 Following UK administration, there is resolution of the thrombus in the UMA as shown in this shallow RAO (A) and RAO-cranial (B) views.

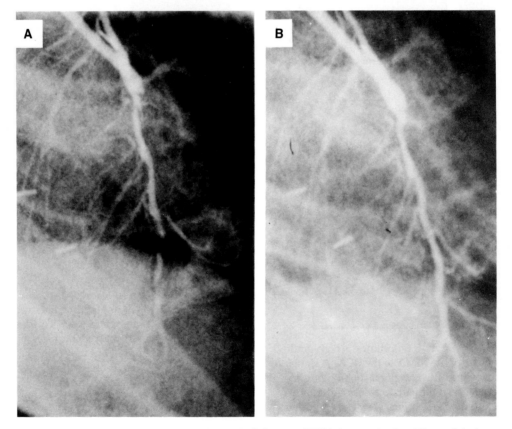

Figure 4-2.9 The filling defect in the LAD following PTCA is seen in the AP-cranial view (A). Following UK, there is also resolution of the distal thrombus (B), which was presumably embolic. To avoid IMA thrombus, one should be certain that the guiding catheter is not "locked" into the IMA ostium, occluding antegrade flow, for prolonged period of time.

Lesion Evaluation in Tortuous Vessels

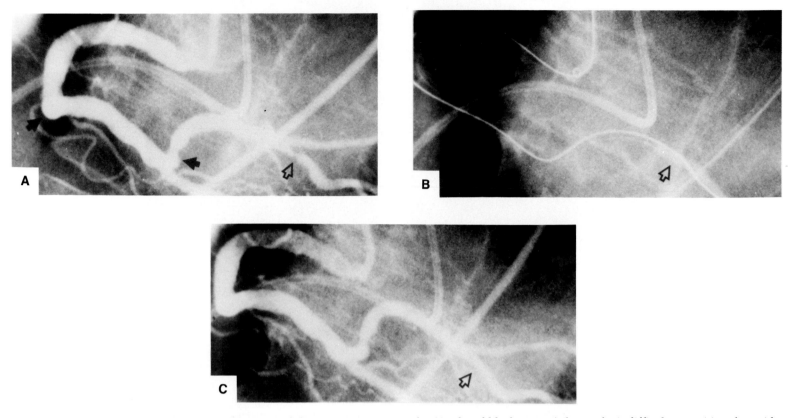

Figure 5-1.5 Note that the RCA is very tortuous and there are two acute angles (A, closed black arrows) that make it difficult to position the guide wire and balloon across the lesion (open arrow) localized in the distal PLB. In (B), a wire has been advanced across the distal lesion but because of the extreme tortuosity, a balloon catheter could not be advanced across the tight stenosis. To maintain lesion access, the guide wire was left across the lesion and a non–over-the-wire balloon catheter (arrow) was advanced in a parallel fashion. The final angiogram shows an excellent result with minimal residual stenosis (C, arrow).

Diffuse Coronary Disease

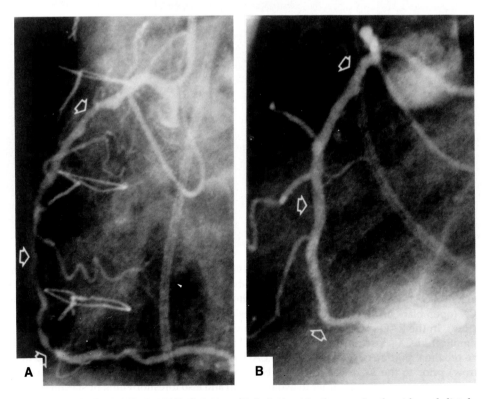

Figure 5-1.6 The LAO view (A) shows multiple lesions in the proximal, mid, and distal portions of the RCA. After successful PTCA, the lateral view (B) reveals marked improvement of the proximal mid- and distal RCA. (Reprinted with permission from Vetrovec GW. Thrombolysis in early transmural myocardial infarction: Feasibility and efficacy. *Postgraduate Medicine* 1985; 77(4):58–67.)

Coronary Ectasia

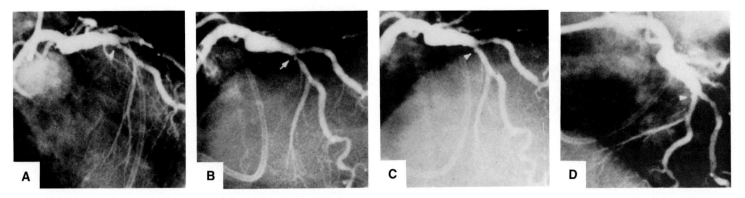

Figure 5-1.7 RAO-cranial (A) and AP-cranial (B) views illustrate a significant stenosis (arrows) just distal to the LAD aneurysm. The post-PTCA result is seen in (C) and (D). AP-cranial (C) and shallow LAO, steep cranial (D) projections illustrate a satisfactory angiographic result without change in the aneurysmal segment.

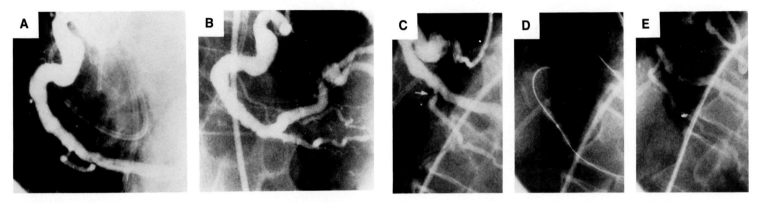

Figure 5-1.8 An ectatic, tortuous RCA with a mid-vessel aneurysm is well visualized in the RAO-caudal (A) and AP-caudal (B) views. An eccentric, proximal PDA stenosis is well visualized in an LAO (30°)-cranial (30°) view (C). This foreshortened view, identifying mid-balloon indentation (D), was helpful to confirm that the balloon was correctly positioned across the lesion. The final angiographic results are again demonstrated in a comparable LAO-cranial view (E).

Vessel Calcification

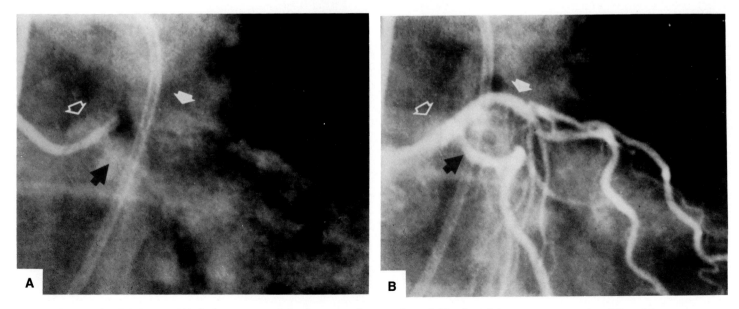

Figure 5-1.9 This RAO view (A), before contrast injection, reveals extensive calcification of the coronary arteries. (The white open arrow identifies calcification in the LMCA while the white closed arrow denotes the LAD outline, and the black arrow identifies calcification in the LCX). In a similar shallow RAO view (B), coronary angiography shows the correlation between the calcifications shown in (A) and the coronary vessels. Fluoroscopic assessment for calcification before contrast injection is important as its presence may potentially determine the PTCA outcome or may affect the alternative nonballoon device used.

Anomalous Coronary Artery

Plaque Morphology

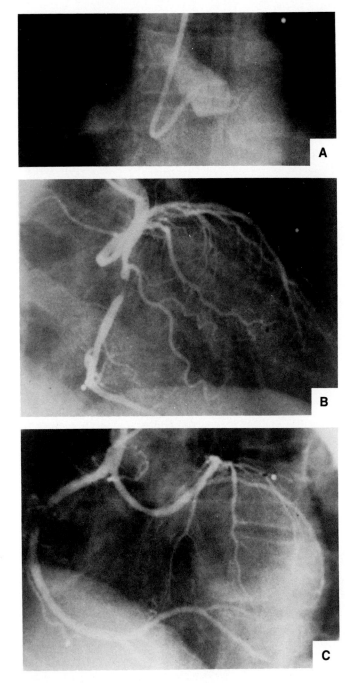

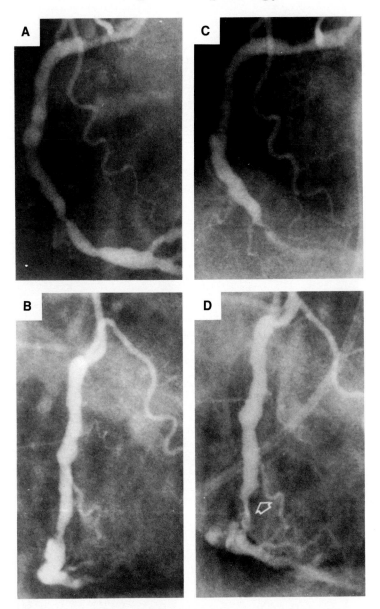

Figure 5-1.10 (A) shows a nonselective injection of the left coronary cusp, identifying no LMCA. In the shallow RAO view (B), injection of the RCA ostium fills the RCA as well as the entire LCA. The LAO-cranial view (C) identifies the essentially common RCA and LMCA origin. The LAD/LCX bifurcation is seen distal to the RCA take off. There is minimal disease in the relatively long LMCA segment. It is important to identify the course of the LM to be certain that it does not traverse between the aorta and the pulmonary artery, increasing the patient's risk for sudden death. In this example, the RCA also has a severe stenosis.

Figure 5-1.11 The matching LAO (A and C) and shallow RAO (B and D) angiograms are separated by a 12-hour interval. In (A) and (B), there is a relatively smooth stenotic lesion in the distal RCA. The comparable (C) and (D) views were taken 12 hours later during an evolving inferior myocardial infarction. In (C), there is a small poststenotic filling defect with slow distal flow. (D) illustrates a new linear dye stain (arrow) not seen in similar views from the earlier angiogram. This linear defect is an angiographic example of a ruptured plaque associated with a thrombotic subocclusion. Careful comparative review of the two angiograms allowed identification of this unusual, but pathophysiologically important finding. (Reprinted by permission from David H. Alpert, MD, et al. Angiographic demonstration of plaque fissure associated with acute coronary occlusion. *American Heart Journal* 117(1):185–186, 1989.)

Intracoronary Thrombus

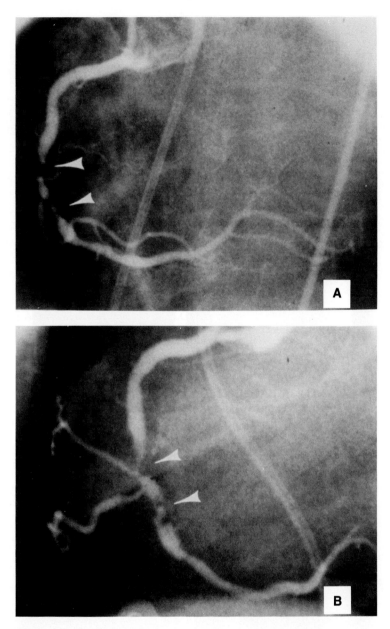

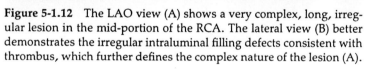

Figure 5-1.12   The LAO view (A) shows a very complex, long, irregular lesion in the mid-portion of the RCA. The lateral view (B) better demonstrates the irregular intraluminal filling defects consistent with thrombus, which further defines the complex nature of the lesion (A).

Intracoronary Thrombolysis

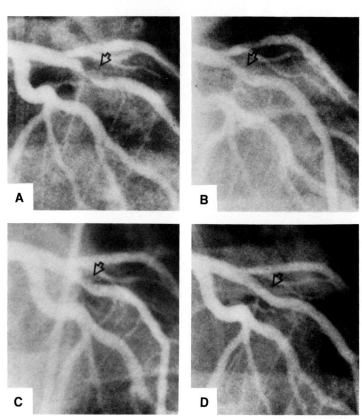

Figure 5-1.17 In the AP-cranial view (A), there is a significant mid-lesion of the LAD with a large intraluminal thrombus identified. In the same view (B), after intracoronary infusion of UK (500,000 units), there is partial resolution of the thrombus (black arrow). Twelve hours after the UK infusion (C), there is persistence of residual thrombus. Following PTCA, there is minimal residual narrowing of the mid-portion of the LAD (D).

Evaluating Bifurcation Branch Lesions

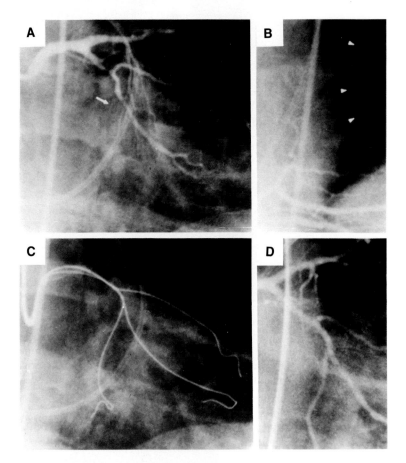

Figure 5-1.18 Pre-PTCA angiography (A) after a recent myocardial infarction with successful thrombolytic reperfusion. There is persistent, severe stenotic disease associated with recurrent postinfarction angina. (A) illustrates a severe marg stenosis with diffuse disease involving the distal marg branches and a suggestion of a third lower branch faintly visualized (arrow) in an RAO projection. (B) is the late phase of an RCA injection in a similar RAO projection, illustrating (three arrows) collateral filling of a low marg branch corresponding to the subtotally occluded segment in the preceding panel. Collateral LCX visualization is frequently easiest in an RAO projection although confirmation of the LCX distribution is best made in an LAO projection. (C) is a shallow RAO view showing three guide wires in each of the branches to allow dilatation of the primary site, while maintaining patency in the branches. Angiographic demonstration of the branch ostium in (A) and the orientation of the third branch in (B) provides the information necessary for successful guide wire placement as shown in (C). The final result, showing all three branches widely patent with minimal residual disease in the primary LCX lesion, is seen in (D).

Evaluating Bifurcation Branch Lesions

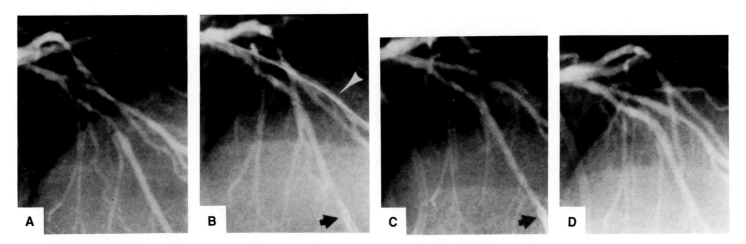

Figure 5-1.19 The AP-cranial view (A) shows a long tubular lesion in the LAD immediately beyond the origin of a diag branch with an ostial lesion. After balloon inflation across both the LAD and diag lesions (B), a test injection is performed with guide wires still across both lesions (arrows). The result appears adequate; however, to better assess each branch separately, the guide wires are sequentially removed from each vessel. In (C), the guide wire is removed from the diag and a test injection is repeated while maintaining guide wire access of the most important vessel (ie, the LAD) (arrow). Finally, in (D), both wires are removed and the angiogram shows an adequate result for both vessels.

Bifurcation Branch Lesions: Balloon Positioning

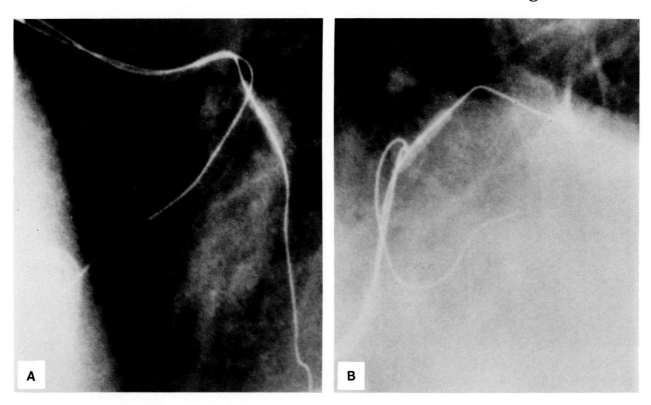

Figure 5-1.20 Effective PTCA of an ostial stenosis requires exact balloon positioning. Careful positioning is particularly important in proximal diag and LAD segments because the balloon may partially inflate in the LMCA, thus blocking LCA flow producing global ischemia. Shown here is balloon inflation identified in an ostial diag lesion during dual wire PTCA of an LAD/diag bifurcation lesion. Position of the inflated balloon across the diag ostium is confirmed by its crossing relationship with the LAD wire seen in the LAO-cranial (A) and particularly in an LAO-caudal view (B).

Bifurcation Branch Lesions: Balloon Positioning

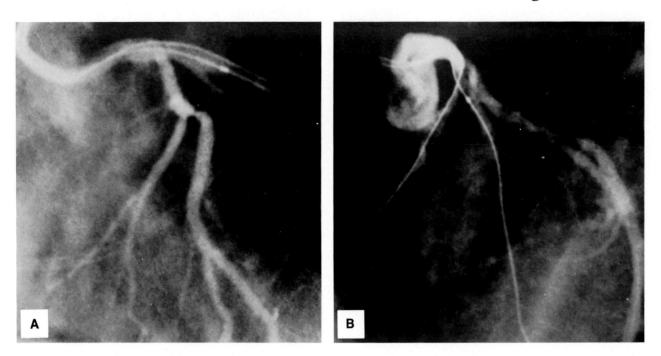

Figure 5-1.21   Another example shown here includes dual guide wire access of a proximal LAD/diag bifurcation lesion. During balloon inflation in the diag, test injections shown in the shallow RAO (A) and LAO-cranial (B) projections confirm the ostial diag balloon position, while demonstrating prompt flow in the LCX. Because of the very proximal diag position, the potential effect of the inflated balloon on LCX flow was uncertain, without contrast test injection particularly in the RAO projection.

Postangioplasty Coronary Dissection

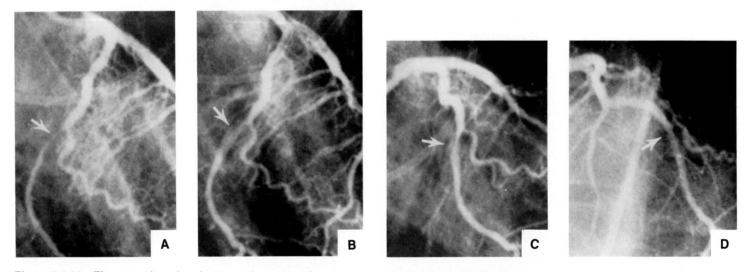

Figure 5-1.22   There is subtotal occlusion at the origin of a second marg branch in the RAO-caudal view (A). After balloon inflation in the RAO-caudal view (B), there is evidence of linear dissection but the lumen of the marg branch is widely patent. A shallow RAO view (C) shows that the dissection involves both sides of the vessel with significant residual luminal narrowing. In the LAO view (D), the lumen is widely patent and the linear dissection is not seen. Thus, unless multiple postprocedure views are obtained, a significant dissection potentially affecting branch flow may not be identified.

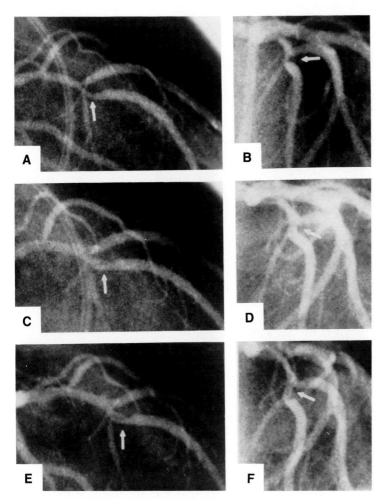

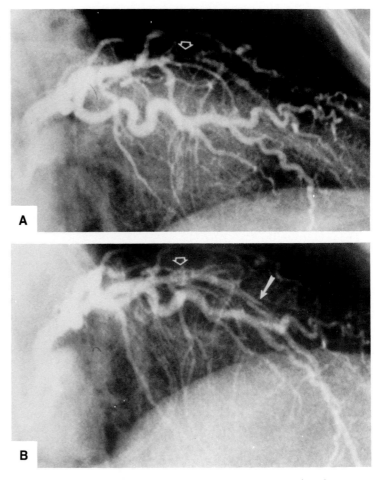

Figure 5-1.23   In the RAO-cranial view (A), there is an eccentric lesion of the LAD after the takeoff of the second diag branch. The AP-cranial view (B) reveals the eccentricity of the stenosis. The immediate post-PTCA angiogram (C and D) shows minimal residual narrowing but a small filling defect that is more obvious in the AP-cranial view (D). Follow-up angiography 48 hours after the PTCA procedure in similar views (E and F) reveals a major intimal dissection with an intraluminal filling defect. Comparable follow-up views are helpful in assessing any progressive adverse outcome from a recent PTCA before proceeding with a second-stage procedure.

Figure 5-1.24   In the RAO-cranial view (A), there is total occlusion in the mid-portion of the LAD. After successful PTCA (B), there is minimal residual narrowing at the primary site (open arrow) but there is a linear dissection distal to the occlusion site (closed arrow) without flow compromise.

Postangioplasty Coronary Dissection

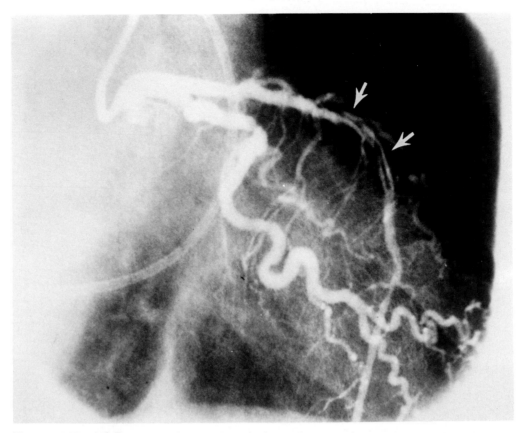

Figure 5-1.25 A follow-up angiogram, 2 weeks later, shows continued patency of the LAD but with persistence of a major intimal dissection.

Healing of Coronary Dissection

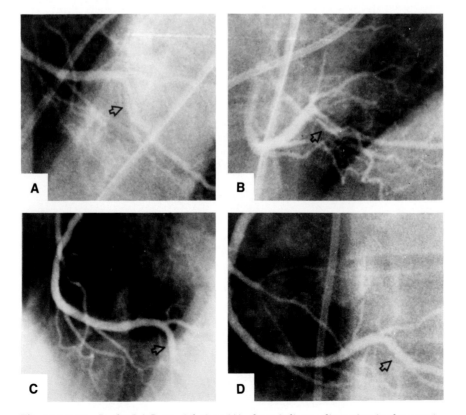

Figure 5-1.26 In the LAO-cranial view (A), there is linear dissection in the proximal portion of the PDA immediately following PTCA. In the shallow RAO view (B), there is even better delineation of the extent of dissection in the proximal PDA. Follow-up angiogram 6 months later shows complete healing of the dissection of the proximal PDA shown in the LAO-cranial (C) and LAO (D) views.

Coronary Tone Variation

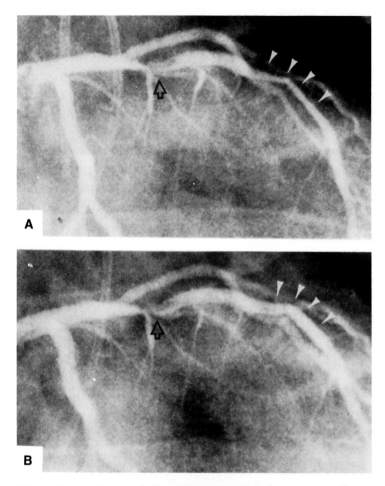

Figure 5-1.27 In the shallow RAO view (A), there is a significant mid-LAD stenosis with a large associated intraluminal thrombus (black arrow). The distal vessel (small white arrows) is diffusely constricted. After intracoronary UK (B), there is mild improvement in the thrombotic LAD stenosis (open black arrow) with marked dilatation of the LAD segment beyond the lesion (white arrows). The vessel size beyond a severe stenosis may be constricted suggesting distal vessel disease. However, by administering nitroglycerin or by improving flow, distal vessel dilatation may result as shown. Thus, failure to recognize potential vessel size and extent of myocardial distribution may adversely affect decisions regarding the need for proximal vessel PTCA. Likewise, recognition of the true vessel size may avert unneeded distal vessel PTCA for presumed diffuse disease.

Angioplasty-Induced Spasm

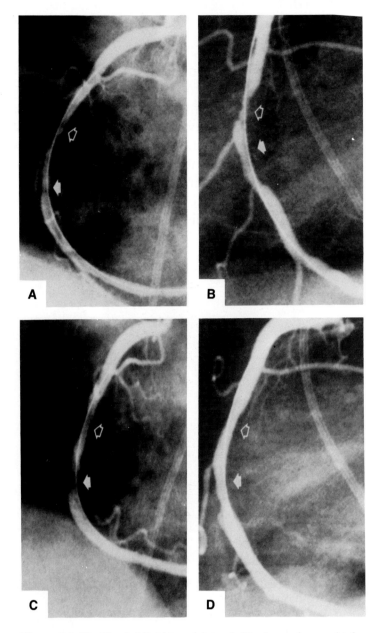

Figure 5-1.28 The LAO (A) and lateral (B) views show a high-grade lesion in the mid-portion of the RCA (open arrow) followed by a mild narrowing (closed arrow). In the LAO view (C), after successful PTCA of the primary lesion (open arrow), the secondary area appears to be more narrowed (closed arrow). However, the smooth nature of the narrowing suggest that this may not be dissection. After the administration of intracoronary nitroglycerin, the lateral view (D) demonstrates resolution of the secondary stenosis, confirming that a significant component of the initial distal stenosis was spasm. (Reprinted by permission from George Vetrovec, MD. Chapter 15. In Carl J. Pepine, MD, et al. *Diagnostic and Therepeutic Cardiac Catheterization.* 1989. Copyright © 1989, the Williams & Wilkins Co., Baltimore.)

Combined Restenosis and Coronary Disease Progression

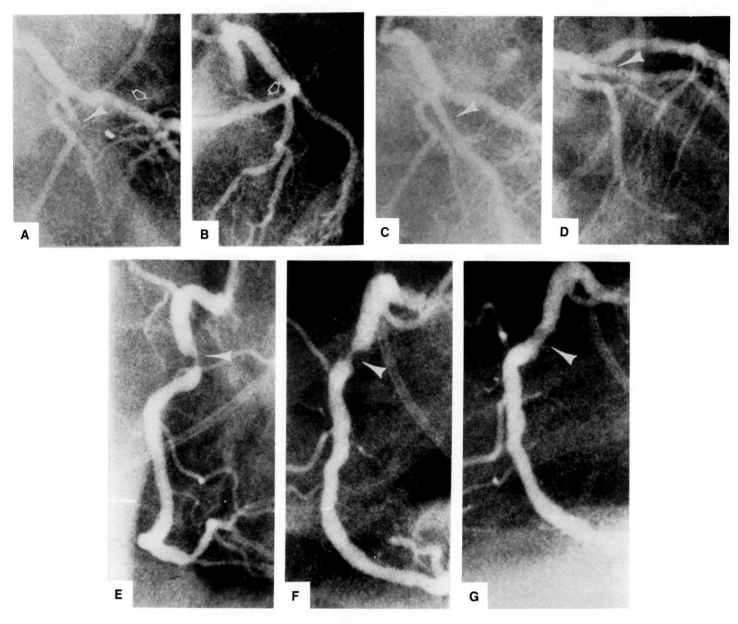

Figure 5-2.4   In the RAO-caudal view (A), there is total occlusion of a marg branch (closed arrow) but there is no significant disease in the proximal portion of the LAD (white arrow). Likewise in the LAO-cranial view (B), there is no significant lesion in the proximal portion of the LAD. After successful PTCA of the totally occluded marg, there is minimal residual narrowing seen in an RAO-caudal view (C). The excellent angiographic result of the marg branch is confirmed in an RAO (15°) view (D). The RCA has a very eccentric proximal lesion in the RAO (E) and lateral (F) views. (G) illustrates the excellent angiographic result post-PTCA during a second-stage procedure.

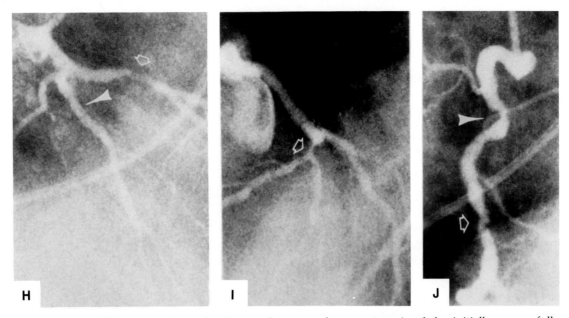

Figure 5-2.4 Follow-up angiography 5 years later reveals no restenosis of the initially successfully dilated marg branch (closed arrow) seen in the RAO-caudal view (H). However, there is significant progression of disease in the proximal portion of the LAD, identified by open arrows in the RAO-caudal (H) and LAO-cranial (I) views. In addition, the RAO (15°) view of the RCA (J) shows partial restenosis of the proximal lesion and a new eccentric stenosis in the mid-portion (open arrow). This sequential angiographic study demonstrates late progression of coronary disease as well as partial restenosis.

Rapid Progression of Coronary Disease

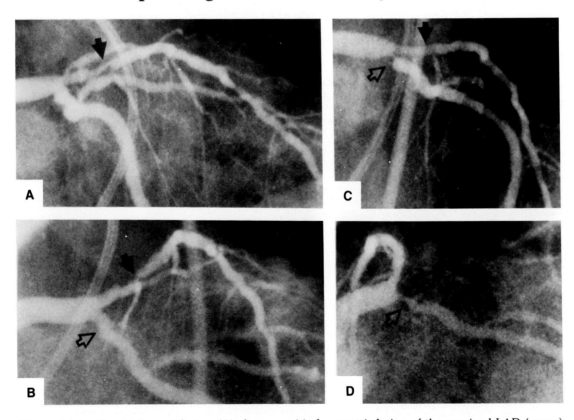

Figure 5-2.5 The RAO-cranial view (A) shows a critical, eccentric lesion of the proximal LAD (arrow) with associated significant narrowing in the mid-portion. The AP-caudal view (B) identifies a significant lesion in the proximal LAD (closed arrow) but demonstrates no significant disease involving the ostium or proximal LCX (open arrow). Four months after successful angioplasty of the LAD, this shallow RAO view (C) shows no restenosis of the LAD (closed arrow), but shows a new high-grade lesion at the ostium of the LCX (open arrow). The ostial LCX lesion is likewise confirmed in an LAO-caudal view (D). This is an unusual example of early recurrent symptoms after PTCA secondary to rapid progression of coronary disease without restenosis.

Late Coronary Disease Progression

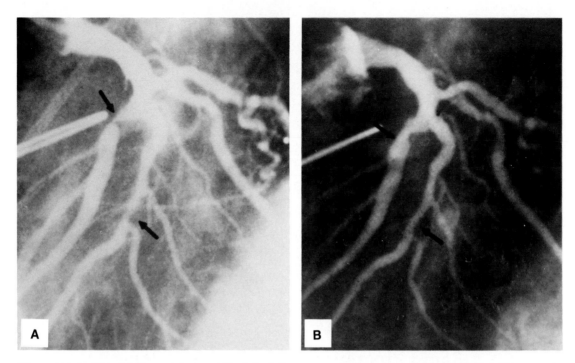

Figure 5-2.6   This LAO-cranial view (A) of the left coronary system demonstrates a 90% LAD stenosis and a significant diag stenosis pre-PTCA in a patient with prior porcine aortic valve replacement. Immediately, post-PTCA (B), left coronary injection shows an excellent diag result with moderate improvement in the LAD.

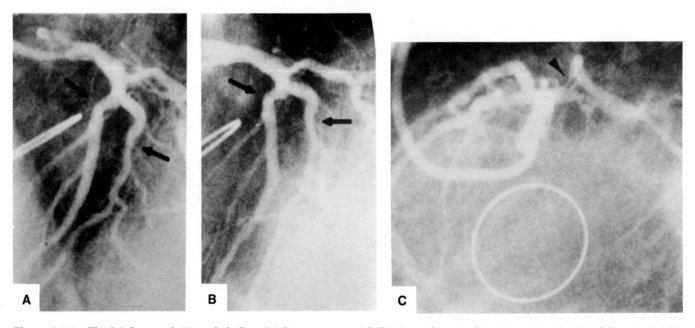

Figure 5-2.7   The LAO-cranial (A) and shallow LAO, steeper cranial (B) views show no late recurrence 8 years following LAD/ diag PTCA (arrows). The ultimate healing of the LAD was improved over the initial post-PTCA results. Note also in (C) that the intermediate marg is now significantly stenotic as shown in an extreme LAO-caudal view, which is excellent for identifying the ostium of an intermediate marg branch. In this particular case, other views were not diagnostic.

5-3 ACUTE CLOSURE

Acute closure is the major cause of urgent bypass surgery for failed angioplasty; however, most patients who develop acute closure can be identified in the laboratory prior to the occurrence of total closure. Repeat angioplasty or utilization of alternative techniques, such as salvage directional coronary atherectomy or prolonged inflation using a perfusion balloon catheter, may ultimately produce an adequate result. To accomplish this goal, it is crucial to recognize the angiographic characteristics of lesions at risk for abrupt closure post-PTCA.

Clinical characteristics for acute closure include recent infarction or unstable angina attributed to the lesion undergoing PTCA. Angiographic features as-sociated with acute closure include lesion-associated thrombus either pre- or post-PTCA, or major or long dissection, particularly with flow compromise. It is important to note that most acute closures occur within 30 minutes after the last inflation. Thus, performing serial angiograms for 10–15 minutes, while a guide wire is maintained across the lesion in high-risk patients or lesions, will identify the majority of patients who have early deterioration of the initial angiographic result and require reintervention to prevent acute closure. By preventing the occurrence of total occlusion, particularly with maintained guide wire access, additional procedures can be performed to achieve an adequate result or to stabilize patients going to urgent bypass surgery.

Figures 5-3.1 to 5-3.8 illustrate recognition and management of potential acute closure.

Spiral Coronary Dissection

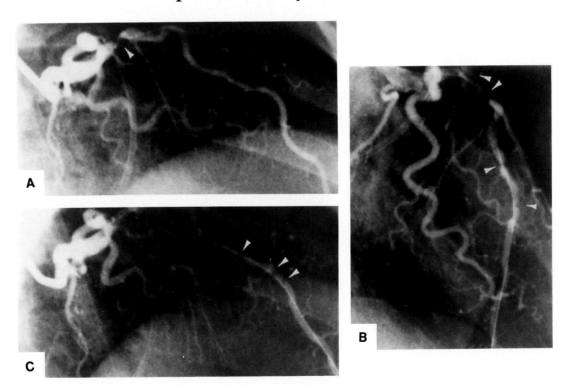

Figure 5-3.1   The RAO-cranial view (A) shows a very eccentric, complex lesion of the proximal portion of the LAD. After the first balloon inflation (B), there is evidence of a significant extraluminal dissection at the primary lesion site as well as extension of the dissection beyond the lesion as shown by the arrows in the mid-LAD segment in this RAO-caudal view. The RAO-cranial view (C) also shows the extension of the spiral dissection to the early distal vessel segment with very irregular, significantly obstructive, negative contrast densities (arrows). Because of the length of this dissection and concern about impending closure the patient was taken to urgent bypass surgery. At the time of surgery, it was noted that the dissection had spiraled down to the apex. The negative defects illustrated in the angiogram presumably included part of the dissection as well as possible associated thrombus. Once the extent of dissection was noted, by maintaining guide wire access and by performing serial angiograms, the patient was able to go to urgent surgery before acute closure and severe ischemia occurred.

Thrombotic Acute Closure

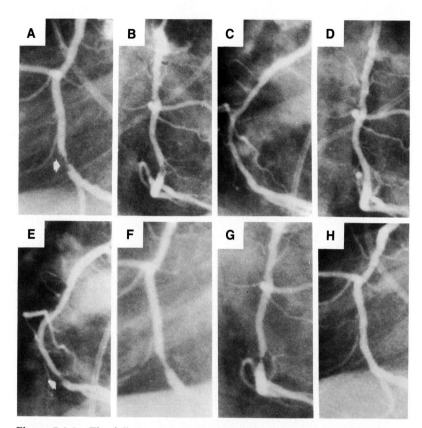

Figure 5-3.2 The following series illustrates the importance of clinical and angiographic lesion assessment in preventing acute closure outside the laboratory. Unstable clinical syndromes, such as unstable angina or myocardial infarction, represent a major clinical risk factor for acute closure during PTCA of the culprit lesion. Lateral (A) and shallow RAO views (B) illustrate a thrombotic irregular lesion in the early distal RCA seen immediately pre-PTCA in a patient with recent accelerated unstable angina pectoris. (C) and (D) illustrate the post-PTCA result in LAO-caudal and shallow RAO projections. There is minimal residual stenosis but significant haziness. The patient was observed because of the recognized clinical and angiographic risks for potential early reclosure. More symmetric but severe early reclosure is seen in multiple projections: LAO (E), lateral (F), and RAO (G) at 10 minutes after the initial successful PTCA. (H) illustrates a lateral view showing the final stable result after repeat angioplasty with prolonged balloon inflations and 15 minutes of in-lab observation that showed no recurrent closure. (Reprinted by permission from George Vetrovec, MD. Chapter 15. In Carl J. Pepine, MD, et al. *Diagnostic and Therapeutic Cardiac Catheterization.* 1989. Copyright © 1989, the Williams & Wilkins Co., Baltimore.)

Extensive Coronary Artery Dissection

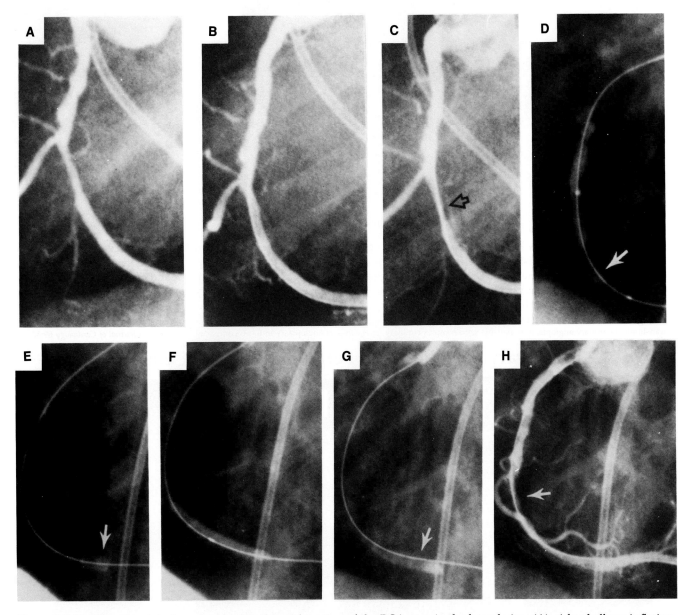

Figure 5-3.3 There is a tubular narrowing in the mid-portion of the RCA seen in the lateral view (A). After balloon inflation, the lateral view (B) shows minimal residual narrowing. The guide wire was maintained in place and after several minutes of observation a test injection shows partial reclosure in the mid-portion of the RCA (C). A perfusion balloon catheter is inflated across the lesion and there is evidence of dye staining distal to the balloon seen in this LAO view (D, arrow). The LAO view (E) shows propagation of the intimal dissection further down the RCA. (F) reveals more distal balloon inflation across the dissection. Following a test coronary injection (G), there is dye stagnation in the false channel due to progression of the spiral dissection. Finally, a repeat angiogram shows persistence of a significant lesion in the mid-portion of the RCA (arrow) as well as distal spiral dissection seen best in an LAO-caudal view (H), which well delineates the mid-distal segment of the RCA.

Antegrade and Retrograde Left
Coronary Dissection

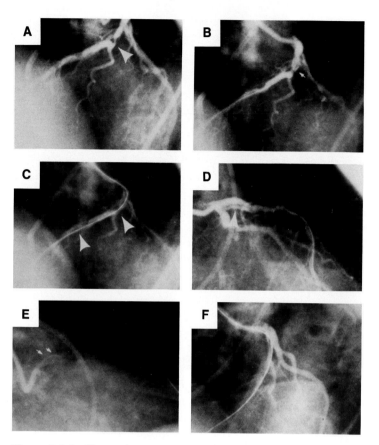

Figure 5-3.8 Shown here is an extensive spiraling dissection from dilatation of an eccentric proximal LAD stenosis seen in the LAO-cranial projection pre-PTCA (A) and immediately after dilatation (B), demonstrating the significant dissection (arrow). Complementary LAO-cranial and shallow RAO views (C and D) illustrate the extent of LAD dissection distally (C) and proximally (D) (arrows). Finally, an RAO-cranial view (E) postinjection shows persistent LM contrast staining (arrows) suggesting LM dissection, which is confirmed by a repeat injection in the LAO-cranial view (F). There is also persistent proximal LAD dissection with impaired distal LAD filling. The recognition of extensive LM dissection precluded further attempts at in-lab stabilization and the patient went to urgent bypass surgery.

5-4 TOTAL OCCLUSION

Interventional management of total occlusion requires preprocedure assessment of the probability of success. Recent acute occlusions, predicted partially by history, by angiographic lesion morphology suggestive of thrombus, and by a beak appearance at the occlusion site, are associated with a higher probability of success. Conversely, chronic, blunt, calcified occlusions, especially with long skip areas, are less suitable for recanalization. Careful assessment of the involved artery as well as collateral filling of the distal vessel in similar views is important to determine the length of the occlusion and the probability of success.

Examples (Figures 5-4.1 to 5-4.6) are presented here that illustrate these concepts.

Recent Total Occlusion: Assessment of Lesion Length

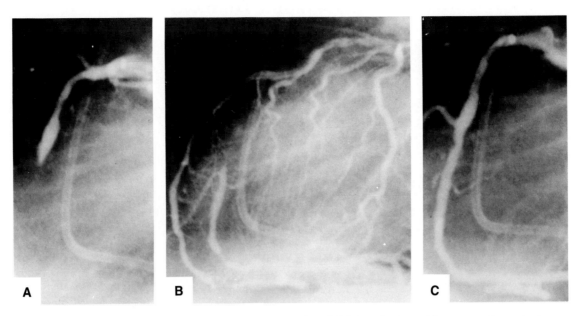

Figure 5-4.1 This lateral projection (A) illustrates total mid-RCA occlusion with a tapered terminal segment consistent with a recent total occlusion. (B) represents the late phase of a lateral LCA injection illustrating marked RCA collateral filling. Comparison of the two injections allows one to assess the actual length of total occlusion, which in this illustration is quite short. (C) shows the final result after successful PTCA. Matching right and left coronary injections in the lateral projection often allows effective assessment of the length of a total mid-RCA occlusion.

Chronic Total Occlusion: Late Collateral Filling

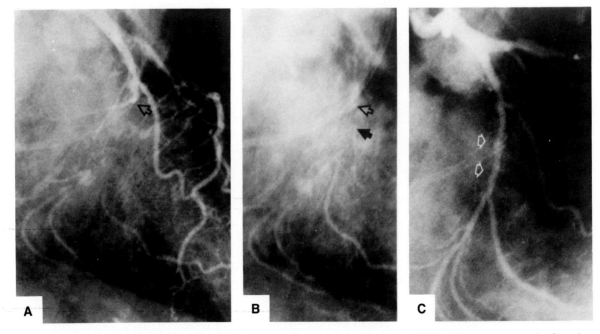

Figure 5-4.2 The RAO-caudal view (A) shows a chronic occlusion of the LCX AV groove vessel after the takeoff of a moderately large marg branch. Although this lesion was successfully dilated, a number of factors predicted a lower probability of success. These factors include the blunt total occlusion (open black arrow) associated with a relatively long skip area as identified by the collateral filling from the antegrade LCA injection. In addition, there is an atrial branch at the point of occlusion that may result in repeated guide wire entry on trying to cross the total occlusion. The collateral filling is well visualized in the RAO-caudal view (B), showing late partial filling of the mid-vessel, which suggests that the occlusion is only moderate in length. Unless a late collateral filling angiogram is obtained, one might be misled by the view in (A) that suggests a much longer extent of occlusion. After successful PTCA of the total occlusion (C), there is no residual narrowing and restoration of brisk antegrade flow.

Chronic Total Occlusion Recanalization: Late Angiographic Follow-Up

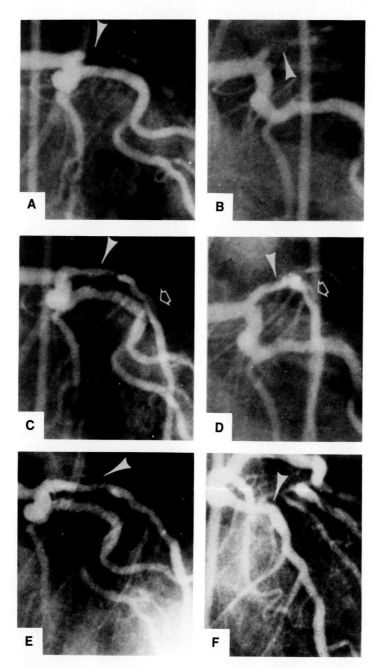

Figure 5-4.3   Shown here is a total occlusion in the proximal portion of the LAD well visualized in a shallow RAO view (A) and in an AP-caudal view (B), which clearly defines the proximal LAD. Note that the arrows indicate the area of total occlusion with early collateral reconstitution of the LAD. After successful dilatation, there is restoration of antegrade flow with mild residual narrowing and modest local dissection (arrow) distal to the previous occlusion site (white open arrow) seen in comparable views (C and D). Repeat angiography 2 years later shows continued patency of the LAD with a minimal residual area of restenosis and complete healing of the intimal dissection. The previous occlusion site of the LAD area is well visualized in a shallow RAO view (E) and an AP-cranial view (F).

Recent Total Occlusion: Embolic Complications

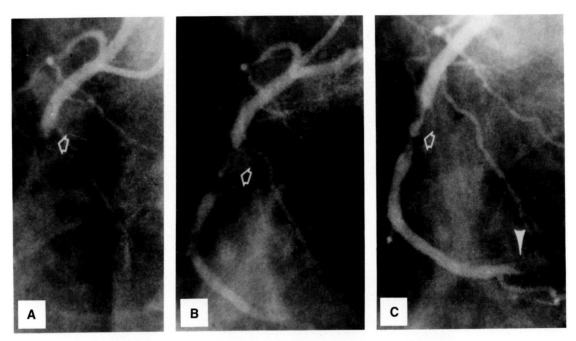

Figure 5-4.4   A proximal blunt early mid-RCA occlusion is shown in a shallow RAO view (A). The distal RCA is not well visualized until after intracoronary UK administration (B), which shows partial recanalization of the RCA with good distal flow but a severely eccentric, thrombotic mid-RCA stenosis. Following further UK administration, there is partial resolution of the thrombotic stenosis in the mid-vessel (C, open arrow), but there is distal occlusion of the RCA (white closed arrow) secondary to embolization from the primary lesion. One risk associated with this complication is that presumably stable distal retrograde collateral flow may be impaired by more distal embolization thus, creating ischemia not present before PTCA.

Change in Collateral Flow Pattern after Angioplasty

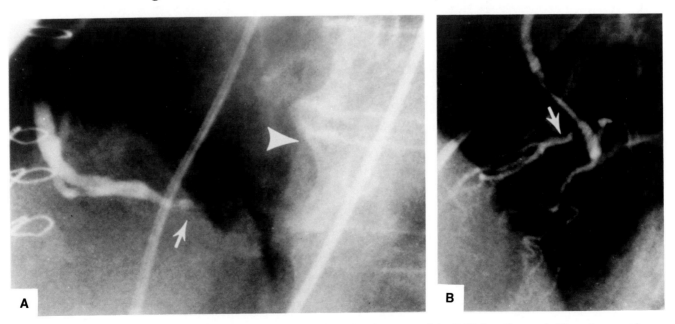

Figure 5-4.5   This LAO view (A) shows a blunt occlusion of the distal portion of the RCA (small arrow). There is no evidence of collaterals to the left coronary system (large arrow). In the LAO-cranial view (B), selected injection in a diagonal vein graft fills the LAD retrograde (arrow).

Change in Collateral Flow Pattern after Angioplasty

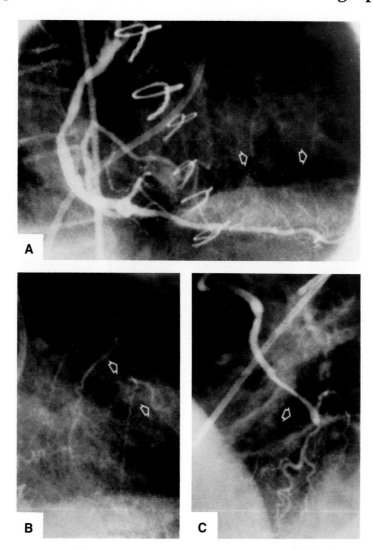

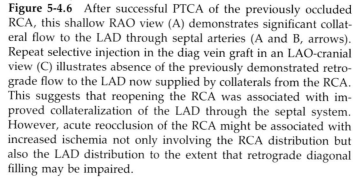

Figure 5-4.6 After successful PTCA of the previously occluded RCA, this shallow RAO view (A) demonstrates significant collateral flow to the LAD through septal arteries (A and B, arrows). Repeat selective injection in the diag vein graft in an LAO-cranial view (C) illustrates absence of the previously demonstrated retrograde flow to the LAD now supplied by collaterals from the RCA. This suggests that reopening the RCA was associated with improved collateralization of the LAD through the septal system. However, acute reocclusion of the RCA might be associated with increased ischemia not only involving the RCA distribution but also the LAD distribution to the extent that retrograde diagonal filling may be impaired.

6

Multivessel Coronary
Artery Disease

Selection of patients for multivessel coronary angioplasty requires identification of persons with the highest probability of success but who are at low risk for complications and for potential restenosis. A person can be considered a favorable candidate if all major affected vessels (lesions) are ideal for dilatation as single arteries, and if no single artery supplies a major myocardial zone through complex collateralization such that acute closure would be associated with severe hemodynamic compromise. Other factors, such as overall LV function, recent myocardial infarction or unstable angina, and the overall risk of bypass surgery, are also important to consider. In addition, length and characteristics of the lesions, to some degree, predict the potential for restenosis; thus, very long lesion or diffuse disease may have a greater risk of recurrence, particularly if it involves several of the arteries being dilated. In order to best make these clinical decisions, ideal angiographic assessment of all involved lesions and vessels is crucial.

Postmyocardial infarction patients require special consideration, particularly because the predominant indication for angioplasty is often a significant residual infarct-related stenosis or occlusion, which is associated with thrombus. Maintaining a stable dilatation result for such lesions is the primary goal and often dictates staging in patients with multiple vessel disease to assure a stable primary result before proceeding to secondary lesions. Again, the assessment of lesion morphology, particularly regarding lesion-associated thrombus, is important in assessing timing and risk of multivessel angioplasty. Left ventriculography is also important in assessing the relative risk of ischemia not only in the distribution of infarct-related vessels but also in the distribution of the other stenotic arteries. To this extent, stable patients are frequently managed with IV heparin for several days to reduce the risk of acute closure associated with PTCA.

Staging patients with multiple vessel disease relates predominantly to the risk of multiple zones of ischemia, which could produce cardiogenic shock in the event of multiple vessel closure. Thus, an angiographically stable primary lesion result is important before proceeding to dilatation of a secondary vessel. Thrombotic lesions or poor initial PTCA results increase the risk of acute closure (see Chapter 5) and the need for staging. Table 6-1.1 and Figures 6-1.1 to 6-1.10 provide suggestions about important issues regarding multiple vessel angioplasty and staging.

Importance of Conus Artery Collaterals

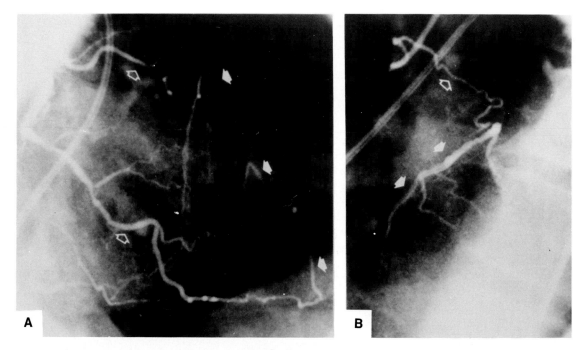

Figure 6-1.3 An RAO view (A) shows a totally occluded RCA in its mid-portion, which provides significant collaterals to the distal LAD as well as faint collaterals to the proximal LAD (closed arrows), predominantly through an RV marg branch (open arrow). Note that on selective injection of the conus artery in an LAO-cranial view (B) there is major filling of the mid- and proximal segments of the LAD, including diag branches. These segments fill substantially better through the conus artery than through the RV branches. This provides assurance regarding dual collateral protection should there be problems in attempting to dilate the RCA unless the conus artery is damaged. In such circumstances, it is important not to obstruct flow to the conus artery during PTCA as this can precipitate ischemia in the LAD distribution. Finally, the conus artery is helpful in considering the alternative possibility of bypass surgery by identifying a high-quality LAD vessel potentially available for graft insertion.

Coronary Collaterals: Multiple Sources

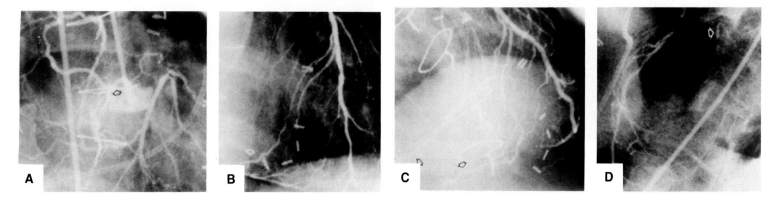

Figure 6-1.4 In these views, total occlusion of the LCX, RCA, and diag vessels are seen. In an RAO view (A) conus collateral filling of the AV groove LCX and marg branches is noted. In an LCA injection in a shallow RAO projection (B), there is marked filling of the mid- and distal PDA through septal collaterals. In addition, there is also collateral filling of the PLB and distal RCA segments from LCA collaterals seen in the RAO-cranial view (C). Finally, the diag is collaterized from the apical LAD as illustrated in an LAO-cranial view (D). Assessing collateral distribution is crucial in determining the safety, feasibility, and strategy for multivessel PTCA.

Multivessel Staging for Coronary Dissection

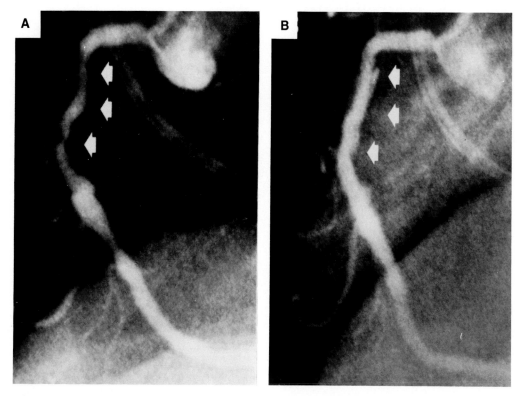

Figure 6-1.5 These lateral views, pre-PTCA (A) and lateral post-PTCA (B), demonstrate a diffuse disease of the mid-RCA. The dilatation was successful but there was a significant degree of localized dissection (B, arrows). The second-stage PTCA was thus deferred to be certain that there was RCA stability before proceeding.

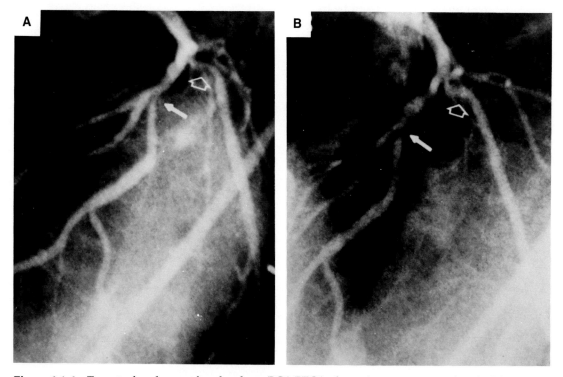

Figure 6-1.6 Twenty-four hours after the above RCA PTCA, the patient was returned to the laboratory. Preliminary angiography indicated no deterioration of the RCA dilatation and, thus, LAD and LAX PTCA was performed. Comparable LAO-cranial views demonstrate the pre-PTCA (A) and post-PTCA (B) results. The LAD stenosis (solid white arrow) demonstrates a favorable result as does the LCX (open white arrow). Assuring that the PTCA site of the large dominant RCA was stable served to enhance the safety of multiple vessel angioplasty.

Multivessel Staging Postmyocardium Infarction

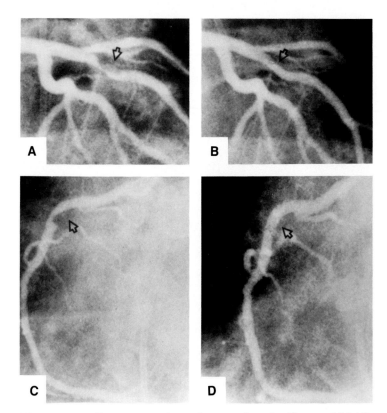

Multivessel Staging for Total Occlusion

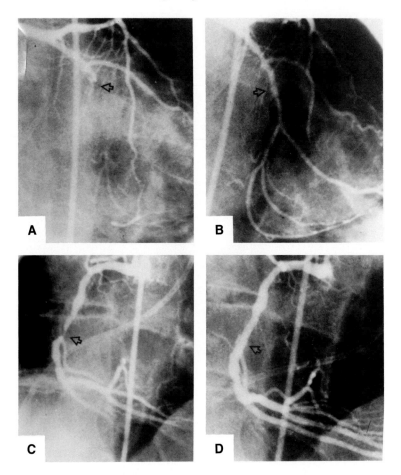

Figure 6-1.7   Coronary angiography reveals a significant mid-LAD lesion with a large intraluminal thrombus (arrow) identified in an AP-cranial view after a nontransmural myocardial infarction (A). Interventional therapy includes intracoronary UK followed by balloon angioplasty, leaving a minimal residual stenosis in the mid-portion of the LAD as seen in a comparable AP-cranial view (B). Five days later, after repeat angiography demonstrating continued patency of the LAD, a second stage procedure was performed. Injection in an LAO view (C) of the RCA demonstrated a significant eccentric proximal stenosis. This lesion was treated with directional atherectomy leaving no significant residual stenosis is seen in a comparable LAO view (D).

Figure 6-1.8   An AP-caudal view (A) demonstrates total occlusion of a large LCX system. There is moderate retrograde LCA collateral filling of only the distal LCX confirming a long segmental occlusion. The occlusion site was successfully traversed and recanalized leaving a mild residual obstruction (B). However, the length of the lesion and the initial total occlusion increased the risk of acute closure, and thus was an indication to defer the second-stage procedure. Twenty-four hours later, angiography demonstrated continued LCX patency and an eccentric severe mid-RCA stenosis that was identified in a shallow RAO view (C). The RCA lesion was successfully treated with directional coronary atherectomy. The final result is seen in a shallow RAO view (D, arrow). Note that there is a small area of dissection associated with the successful atherectomy.

Multivessel Staging: Clinical Factors

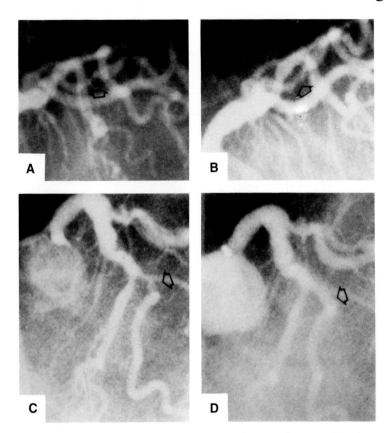

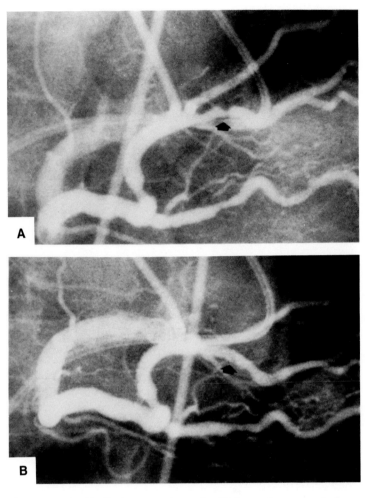

Figure 6-1.9 Shown here is an extremely complex, overlapping coronary anatomy, which required multiple carefully individualized views to identify the lesions. An LAO-caudal view (A) demonstrates a significant lesion arrow in the proximal segment of a high marg branch. In the same view (B), the post-PTCA angiogram demonstrates marked improvement at the dilated site. The LAO-cranial projection (C) was utilized to identify a severe and complex lesion in the proximal portion of a large diag branch, which was also successfully dilated at the same stage as shown in a comparable view (D). However, because of the complexity and duration of the procedure, the amount of contrast required and the presence of some residual haziness suggesting dissection or thrombus in the diag branch, PTCA of the PLB was deferred to a second stage.

Figure 6-1.10 Preliminary angiography 24 hours later revealed no deterioration in the diag and LCX marg PTCA sites. PTCA of the mid-PLB stenosis was then successfully performed as shown in this RAO view (A-pre-PTCA, B-post-PTCA).

7

Nonballoon Interventions

7-1 LASER BALLOON ANGIOPLASTY

The laser balloon concept utilizes laser thermal heating of the artery to provide stability in non-ideal results following standard balloon angioplasty, particularly in the setting of impending or actual acute closure. The technique is effective and often provides a "cast-like" vessel segment after the treatment. The risk of urgent surgery is reduced but the possibility of early restenosis seems to be enhanced. Figure 7-1.1 and 7-1.2 are examples of this technology.

Excimer Laser Recanalization: Native Vessel

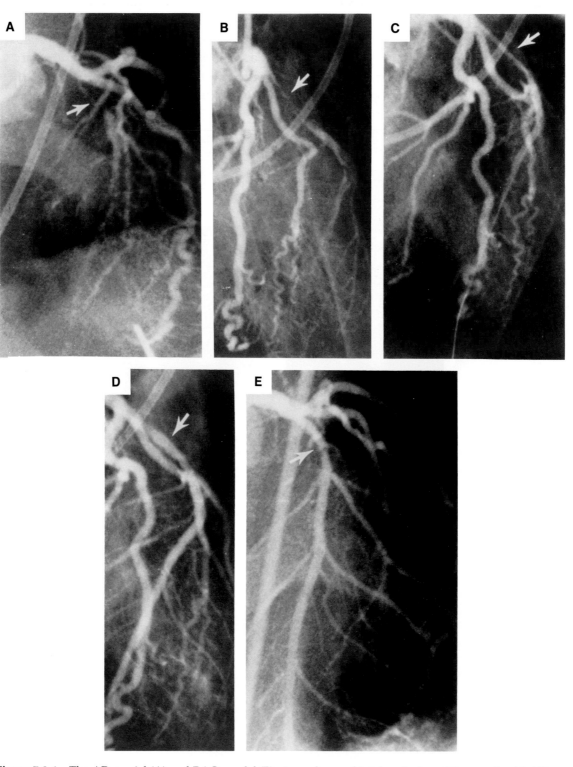

Figure 7-2.1   The AP-cranial (A) and RAO-caudal (B) views show subtotal occlusion of the proximal LAD with an apparent recanalized channel and late collateral filling of the vessel. After passage of an Excimer laser catheter, there is restoration of antegrade flow seen in the RAO-caudal view (C). After laser debulking, adjunctive balloon angioplasty was performed. The final result is seen in an RAO-caudal (D) and an AP-cranial (E) view, illustrating an excellent angiographic result.

Excimer Laser Recanalization: Ostial Vein Graft

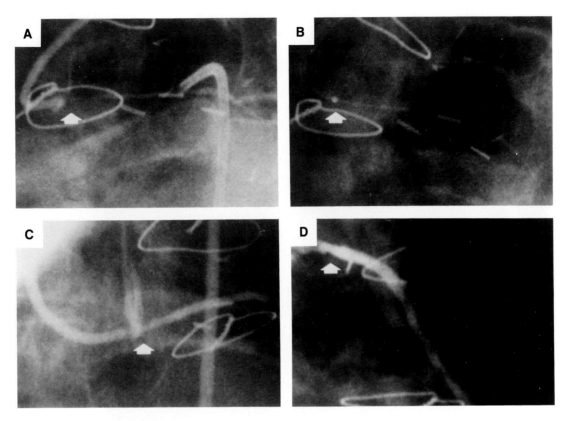

Figure 7-2.2   (A) illustrates a subtotal occlusion vein graft involving the ostium and a long proximal segment of a vein graft. (B) demonstrates the guide wire successfully passed across the lesion and the Excimer laser catheter (arrow) at the ostium. (C) shows minimal residual narrowing at the ostium and proximal vein graft segments following combined Excimer laser and balloon angioplasty. (D) is a 6-month follow-up angiogram showing healing without restenosis of the ostium and proximal segments of the graft. Angiography, in all instances, requires careful seating of the guiding catheter or diagnostic catheter to provide effective injection without damaging the ostium, particularly in the immediate post-PTCA angiograms when the ostium has been dilated.

Excimer Laser Coronary Dissection

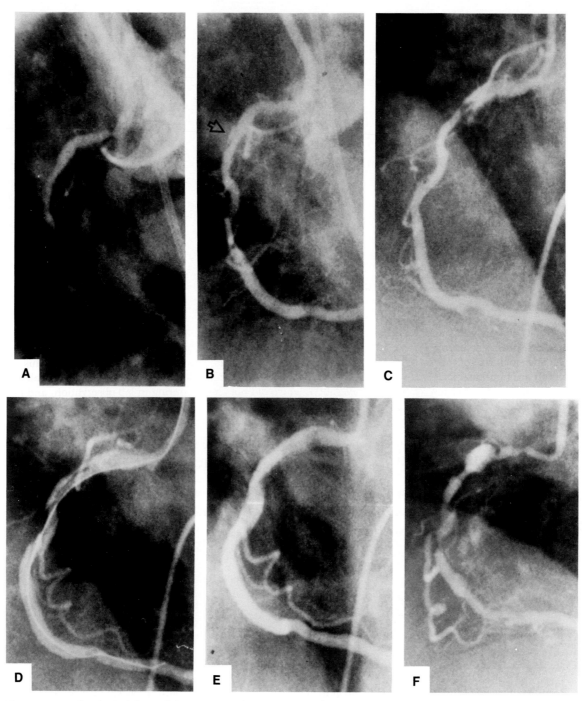

Figure 7-2.6 In the LAO-caudal view (A), there is a critical RCA ostial lesion. After successful ELCA with adjunctive balloon angioplasty, there is minimal residual narrowing at the ostium of the RCA in a similar LAO-caudal view (B). However, there is a dissection cap at the proximal portion of the RCA, which prompted in-lab sequential angiographic follow-up. (C) illustrates the importance of such follow-up as the dissection progressed to subacute closure. The RCA was successfully retraversed with the guide wire. Following repeat balloon inflation there is marked extension of the spiral dissection from the ostium to the mid-portion of the RCA (D). After prolonged perfusion balloon inflation, there is marked improvement in the luminal diameter of the RCA with restoration of brisk antegrade flow (E). However, repeat angiography 3 months later (F) shows multiple lesion in the proximal and mid-portion of the RCA with aneurysmal formation in the proximal segment as well.

7-3 DIRECTIONAL CORONARY ATHERECTOMY

Directional coronary atherectomy provides an excellent angiographic result in a majority of procedures, but is generally limited to more proximal, larger vessel lesions. Thus, angiographic anatomic considerations include assessing the eccentricity, the length (shorter are more suitable), and the proximal location of the lesions. Associated disease beyond the primary lesion may be at risk for nose cone injury and should be evaluated carefully. In addition, the presence of significant calcification makes DCA less ideal. Thus, angiographic assessment of lesion characteristics as well as secondary distal vessel disease is important in the selection of the most suitable candidates for DCA. Finally, assessment of the ostial and proximal vessel size is important because of the need for larger guiding catheters with this device. Figures 7-3.1 to 7-3.5 illustrate these concepts.

Directional Coronary Atherectomy: Lesion Morphology

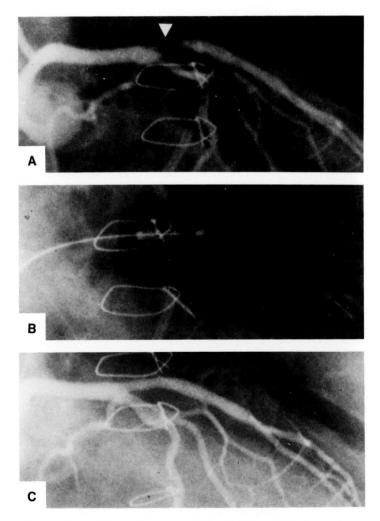

Figure 7-3.1 Shown here are similar RAO-cranial views of the proximal LAD segment beyond a long LMCA illustrating an eccentric LAD stenosis (A, arrow) treated by DCA. (B) shows the atherectomy device across the lesion. DCA is particularly useful in the management of eccentric disease and is frequently associated with a better angiographic result (C) than might have been achieved with balloon angioplasty.

Directional Coronary Atherectomy: Assessing Feasibility

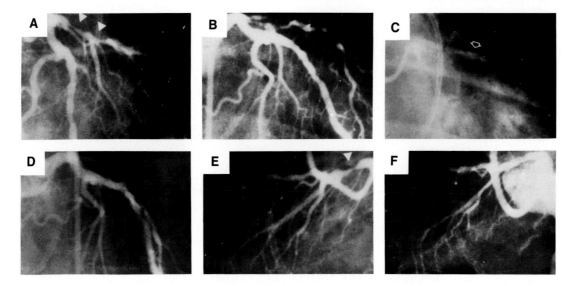

Figure 7-3.2   This case illustrates complex, diffuse proximal and early mid-LAD lesions treated with a combination of DCA (proximal lesion) and PTCA (mid-lesion). The lesions and their relationship to the large septal perforator are well outlined and separated from overlying high LCX branches in RAO-caudal (A) and AP-caudal (B) views. A shallow RAO view (C) illustrates vessel calcification (arrow) seen prior to contrast injection, which was particularly evident in the area of the secondary lesion. The calcification was visualized fluoroscopically prior to any contrast injection excluding the possibility of dye staining as a cause of the hazy white, unopacified vessel wall markings. Furthermore, an AP-cranial view (D) failed to demonstrate the presence of calcification during injection.

The mid-calcification, tortuosity, and mild, late mid-vessel irregularity made DCA unfavorable for the mid-stenosis. Thus, DCA was utilized for the proximal lesion only while balloon angioplasty was utilized for the mid-lesion. (E) and (F) illustrate the proximal lesion in the superlateral view (LAO 110°) pre- and post-DCA. Use of an extreme LAO view eliminates foreshortening of the very proximal LAD segment that often occurs in a standard lateral projection. The addition of minor cranial or caudal angulation may be necessary to avoid overlap of superior diag or marg branches. This example of proximal LAD stenosis lengthening illustrates better lesion morphology assessment pre- and postintervention by specific view selection.

Directional Coronary Atherectomy: Result in an Eccentric Lesion

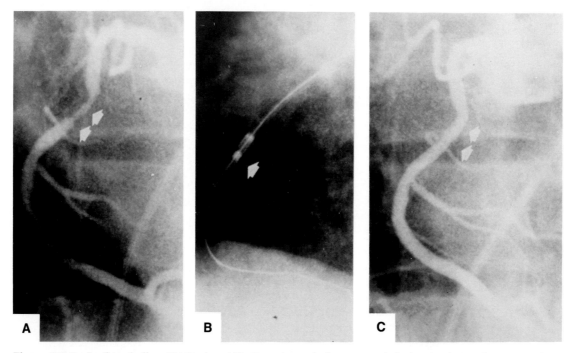

Figure 7-3.3   In this shallow RAO view (A), there is a tubular, eccentric lesion in the mid-portion of the RCA. The DCA device is positioned across the lesion (B). Note how the vessel has been straightened by the device. Post-PTCA, there is a minimal residual lesion in the mid-portion of the RCA (C).

Directional Coronary Atherectomy: Distal Spasm

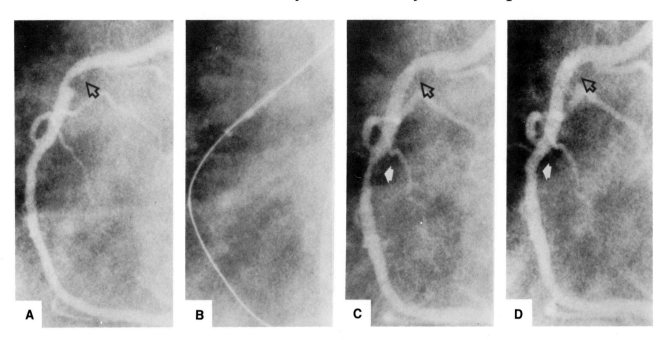

Figure 7-3.4   In the LAO view (A), there is an eccentric, significant lesion in the proximal RCA (arrow). The DCA device is positioned across the lesion (B). In the same LAO view (C), there is excellent angiographic result at the primary DCA site with minimal residual narrowing. However, there is a new symmetric stenotic lesion in the mid-portion of the RCA (white arrow). After intracoronary administration of nitroglycerin, there is resolution of the spasm in the mid-RCA (white arrow), and again, minimal residual lesion is noted at the primary DCA site (D).

Directional Coronary Atherectomy: Local Dissection

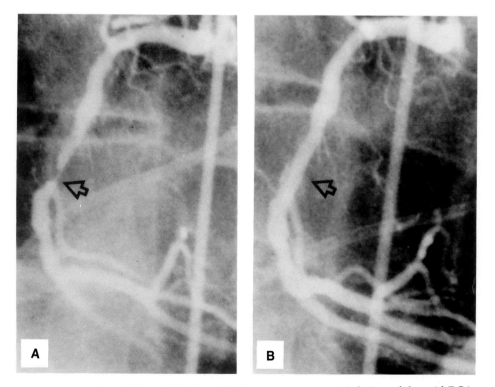

Figure 7-3.5   The shallow RAO view (A) shows a very eccentric lesion of the mid-RCA. After successful DCA (B), there is only very mild residual narrowing but a localized intimal dissection is seen without flow compromise.

7-4 ROTATIONAL CORONARY ATHERECTOMY

Rotational atherectomy technology is effective for diffuse non-ideal balloon lesions, particularly in calcified or smaller distal vessels. In general, however, adjunctive balloon angioplasty is required to manage larger vessels because of size disproportion between the relatively small burr and the larger vessel segments treated with the device. In addition, adjunctive PTCA is utilized to treat coronary spasms that occur frequently following RA. The spasm can be identified by careful angiographic assessment during the procedure and treated with nitrates or balloon inflation. Preprocedure assessment includes choosing lesions in vessels that do not provide the sole remaining myocardial blood supply. This can be important because transient myocardial ischemia may occur as a consequence of embolic particulate matter from the device, causing a *no reflow phenomenon*.

The following examples (Figures 7-4.1 and 7-4.2) illustrate some of these concepts.

Rotational Atherectomy

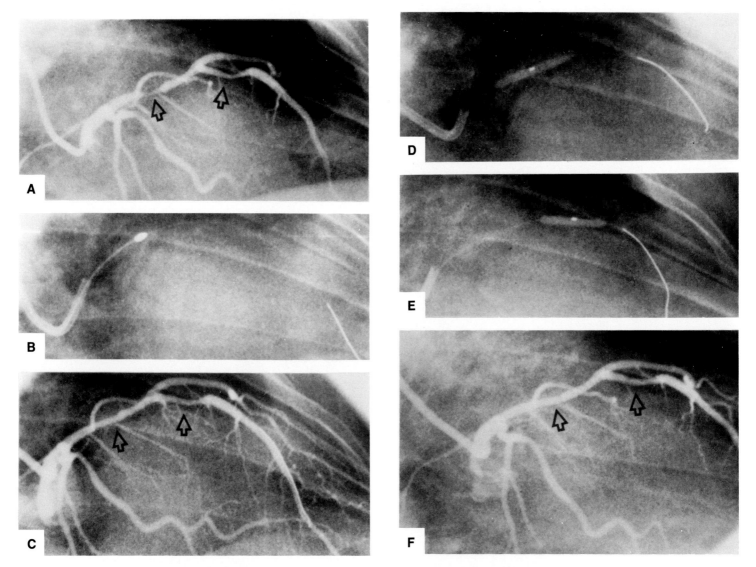

Figure 7-4.1 The RAO-cranial view (A) shows two tubular narrowings in the proximal and mid-portion of the LAD. The RA device is positioned in the first LAD lesion (B). After a single pass of the device, there is marked improvement of both lesions in the LAD (C). Comparable RAO-cranial views show balloon inflation at low pressure in the proximal (D) and mid-lesions (E). The final angiogram shows marked improvement of both lesions in the RAO-cranial view (F).

Rotational Atherectomy: Coronary Spasm

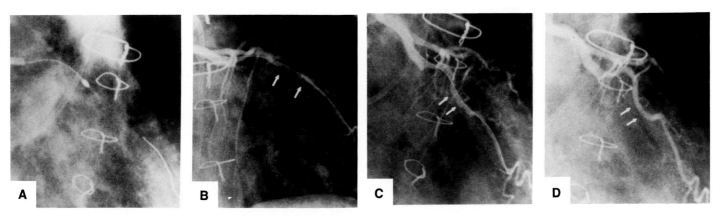

Figure 7-4.2 This RAO-caudal view (A) demonstrates the RA device as it is positioned in the proximal segment of a high marg branch. Following removal of the device, there is angiographic evidence of coronary spasm distal to the RA site (arrows) demonstrated in a shallow RAO view (B). The distal spasm is also seen as a series of focal filling defects in an RAO-caudal view (C). Finally, after withdrawal of the guide wire and administration of intracoronary nitroglycerin there is complete resolution of the coronary spasm (D).

7-5 INTRACORONARY STENTS

Indications for intracoronary stenting include acute vessel closure as well as primary dilatation of focal lesions with the goal of reducing late restenosis. Lesions considered for stent implantation should be fo-cal, optimally requiring a single stent. During the stent placement, careful angiography is crucial to assure proper placement of the stent across the lesion. Later subacute complications of the stent implantation include partial or complete thrombotic closure, which requires either thrombolytics or secondary PTCA. The following examples (Figures 7-5.1 and 7-5.2) illustrate several of these features.

Intracoronary Stent Placement: Angiographic Assessment

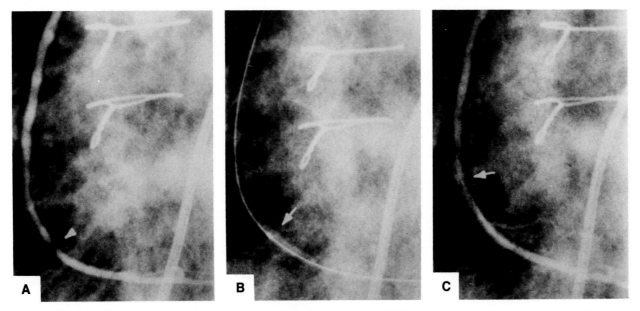

Figure 7-5.1 (A) shows a discrete right vein graft lesion (arrow). (B) illustrates stent deployment during balloon inflation. The final angiographic result (C) reveals mild vein graft dissection at the superior stent border (arrow).

Intracoronary Stent: Subacute Thrombosis

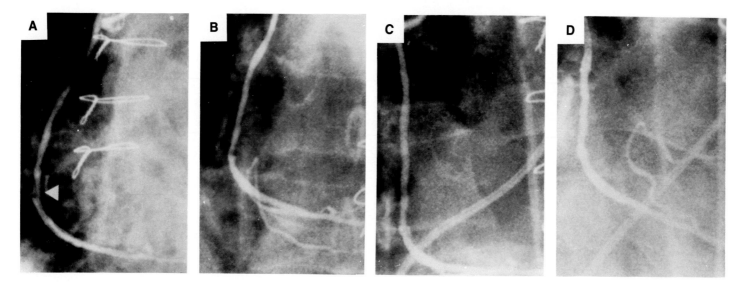

Figure 7-5.2   Two weeks following stent implantation, repeat angiography for unstable angina shows a thrombotic (filling defect) partially occlusive lesion at the superior stent border seen in the LAO (A, arrow) and RAO (B) views. (C) demonstrates thrombus resolution after an overnight intragraft UK infusion. (D) illustrates an excellent final result after adjunctive PTCA.

8

Complications

Complications are undesirable; however, a variety of adverse events are inherent to interventional technology. Thus, operators must always be cognizant of the specific risks involved for each procedure and must always weigh the risks and/or benefits of a possible intervention versus other therapies. Complications of varying severity and consequence include distal embolization, guide wire fracture, and coronary vessel perforation along with acute and subacute closure (Chapter 5-3) and coronary dissection (Chapter 5-1). Early recognition of complications is crucial. Appropriate management may simply require a prolonged in-lab observation to confirm stability of the lesion or may require further intervention or even bypass surgery.

8-1 CORONARY EMBOLIZATION

Coronary embolism is the result of the fragmentation of an existing intracoronary thrombus or the development of a new equipment- or lesion-associated thrombus. Primary equipment-associated thrombus and in situ thrombus, providing that effective anticoagulation and catheter flushing are maintained, are rare. Most often, disruption of a lesion-associated thrombus, which occurs during guide wire or balloon catheter manipulation, results in distal emboli of clot material, producing sludging and poor run-off e.q. to a no reflow phenomenon.

The purpose of angiography is to identify the risk or the consequences of an embolic event. High-quality angiography enhances recognition of pre-PTCA lesion-associated thrombus. Such recognition may affect decisions about the feasibility and the timing of intervention as well as the need for intra-coronary thrombolysis.

An important potential cause of post-PTCA angina is branch or distal vessel embolization, particularly in the setting of a favorable angiographic result of the primary lesion. Meticulous comparison of pre- and post-PTCA angiograms for missing or slow-filling distal vessel segments or branches is important in evaluating the significance of postintervention ischemia.

Figures 8-1.1 to 8-1.4 address specific embolic complications while other sections in the text emphasize lesion morphology related to local thrombus and the impact of intracoronary UK in routine angioplasty.

Intracoronary Thrombus Fragmentation

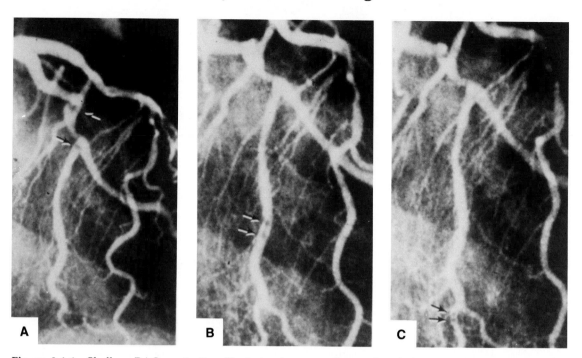

Figure 8-1.1 Shallow RAO projection illustrates fragmentation and embolization of an intracoronary filling defect during the first coronary injection in a patient with recent unstable angina attributed to an LCX lesion. In (A), the top arrow indicates the lesion-associated thrombus with an initial fragment (lower arrow) embolism. The subsequent panels (B and C) illustrate two embolic fragments as they progress down the coronary artery during later frames of the same coronary injection. This illustrates the embolic potential of an intracoronary thrombus, which may occur either spontaneously or in the thrombolytic setting. (Reprinted by permission from George Vetrovec, MD, et al. Intracoronary thrombus in syndromes of unstable myocardial ischemia. *American Heart Journal* 102:1202–1208, 1981.)

Intracoronary Embolus

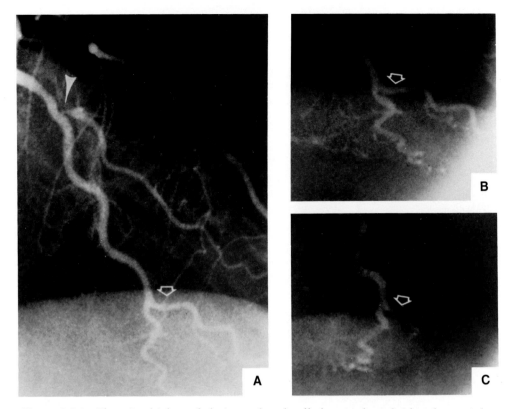

Figure 8-1.2 There is a high-grade lesion at the takeoff of a marg branch (closed arrow) that is seen in the shallow RAO view (A). Note a patent distal marg branch (white open arrow). (B) shows a close-up of the patent small distal branch (open arrow). During attempted PTCA, the marg branch was unable to be cannulated with a guide wire because of marked tortuosity of the proximal LCX. Subsequently, the patient experienced mild chest discomfort. Initial test injection showed patency of the target marg branch, but careful analysis of the angiogram demonstrated embolic occlusion of the small distal marg branch (white open arrow) in this same shallow RAO view (C). Careful comparative angiographic assessment of all vessel segments, pre- and post-PTCA, is useful to exclude possible embolus-induced ischemia.

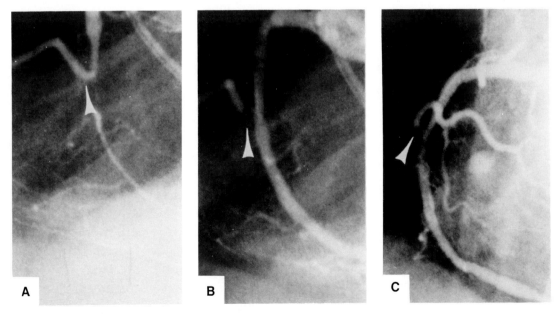

Figure 8-1.3 Subtotal RCA occlusion can be seen in this lateral view (A). The arrow illustrates patency of a modest-sized RV branch. Following successful angioplasty, recanalization of the RCA is demonstrated in the lateral (B) and shallow LAO (C) views. Though the native RCA is widely patent, there is now a thrombotic subocclusion in the ostium of the previously patent RV branch. This illustrates a circumstance in which branch embolization or thrombus may produce ischemic symptoms in the face of an otherwise satisfactory, primary PTCA result.

Intracoronary Embolus

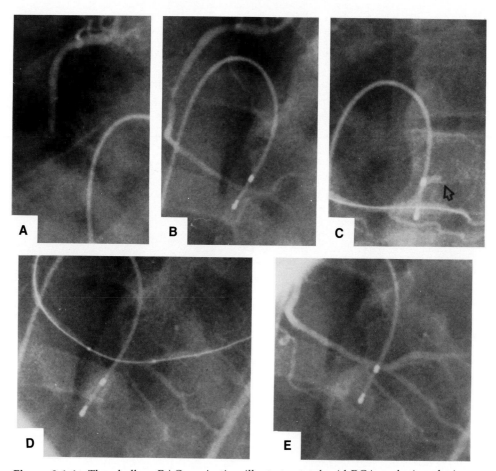

Figure 8-1.4 The shallow RAO projection illustrates total mid-RCA occlusion during an evolving inferior wall myocardial infarction treated with primary PTCA because of contraindication to thrombolysis. The shallow LAO view (A) illustrates total acute occlusion with hazy, blunt, irregular margins (arrow). An AP view (B) illustrates recurrent local thrombus after initial, successful recanalization of the RCA. An LAO view (C), taken minutes later, illustrates an embolic occlusion of the PLB (arrow) with the guide wire positioned in a very low PLB segment. To avoid thrombolysis, the guide wire was steered into and across the embolic PLB occlusion, and a balloon catheter was utilized to fragment and recanalize the vessel (D). The final post-PTCA result is seen in an AP view (E), showing successful distal recanalization.

8-2 MAIN STEM CORONARY ARTERY DISSECTION

Proximal major coronary artery dissection is a serious complication frequently producing severe ischemia. The most frequent cause of ostial or proximal LMCA and RCA dissection is guiding catheter trauma. Routine 8 Fr guiding catheters, though usually constructed with soft tips, still have the potential to produce serious coronary damage. Factors that contribute to the increased risk of catheter-induced coronary dissection during PTCA include (1) the firmer shaft and nontapered tip of guiding catheters compared to diagnostic catheters, (2) the frequent need for special angioplasty curves, and (3) the deep engagement of the guiding catheter for support. Furthermore, newer techniques, such as directional atherectomy and stent placement, utilize larger and sometimes stiffer guiding catheters to deliver the devices. These techniques further increase the risk of coronary dissection, particularly in the setting of small or diseased coronary ostia. Thus, pre-PTCA angiography is important to assess coronary ostial size and possible local disease that may increase the incidence of guiding catheter trauma. Angiography is also important to rapidly assess the presence and the extent of dissection, in case it occurs either as a result of guiding catheter trauma or by retrograde propagation from balloon or device manipulation. Early recognition allows for prompt management, through the use of perfusion devices, stents, or urgent bypass surgery.

Figures 8-2.1 to 8-2.5 illustrate the role of angiography in diagnosis and management of this complication.

Ostial Right Coronary Dissection

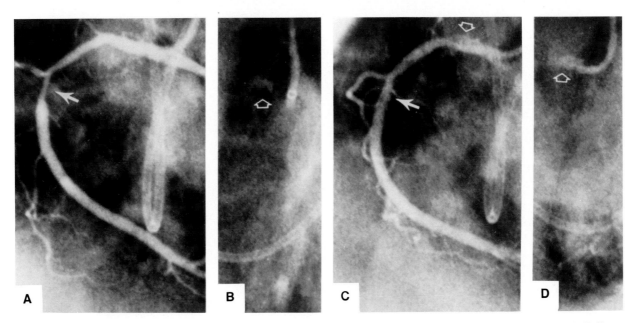

Figure 8-2.1 This is a shallow LAO-cranial view (A), demonstrating a significant mid-RCA stenosis (arrow). Following an initial series of RCA injections, there is late contrast staining in the RCA ostial area seen in an AP view (B). Following successful PTCA of the mid-RCA (closed arrow), the staining is again seen in the LAO-cranial view (C). Evidence of proximal RCA dissection (open arrow) at the tip of the diagnostic catheter is seen as a persistent postinjection stain (D). In the absence of symptoms, ischemia, or acute in-lab deterioration, the patient was managed medically.

Ostial Right Coronary Dissection

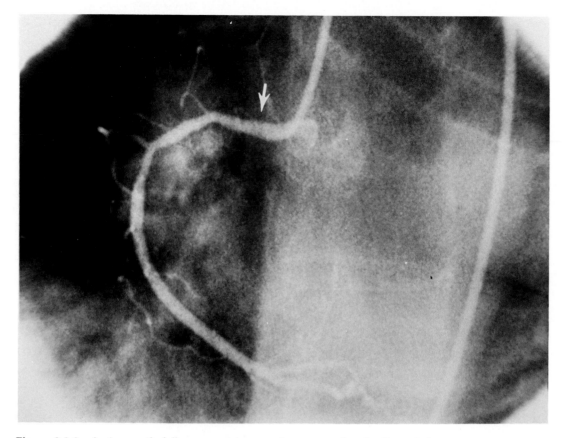

Figure 8-2.2 A six-month follow-up angiogram shows complete healing of the ostial dissection as previously reported. If the initial dissection remains stable, without flow compromise, complete healing usually occurs.

Left Main Retrograde Dissection

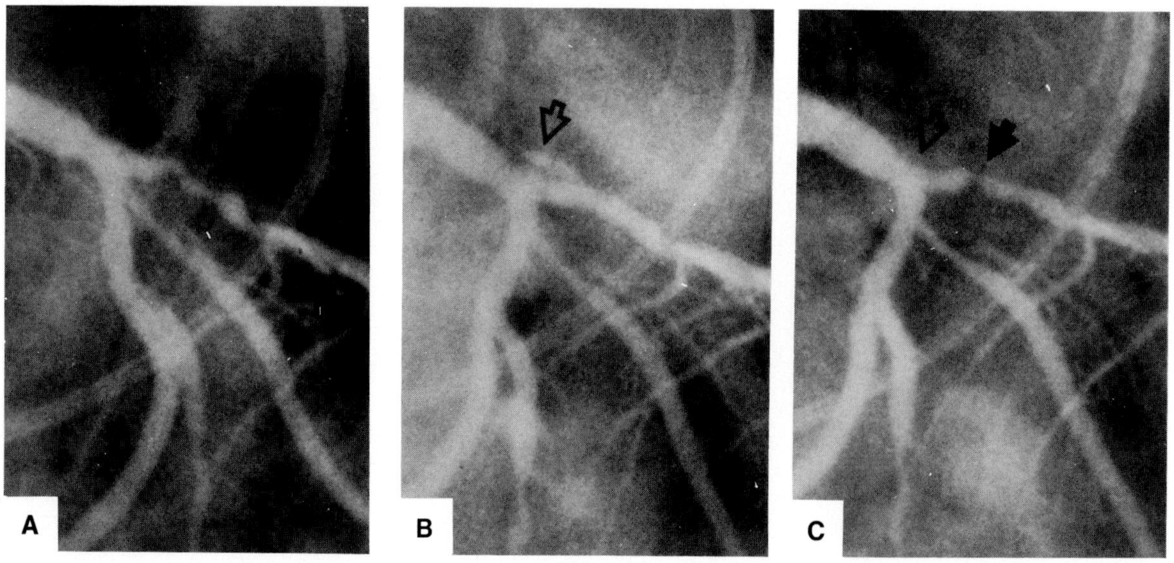

Figure 8-2.3 There is a long, tubular, very proximal lesion in the LAD seen in the RAO-caudal view (A). After balloon inflation (B), there is minimal residual narrowing of the primary PTCA site. However, a balloon-induced dissection propagated retrograde to the distal LMCA. Because no deterioration occurred after prolonged in-lab observation, no additional intervention was performed. Four months following PTCA, a repeat angiogram (C) showed complete healing of the LMCA dissection (open arrow) with a more discrete restenotic lesion of the LAD (closed arrow) illustrated in the RAO-caudal view.

Catheter-Induced Left Main Dissection

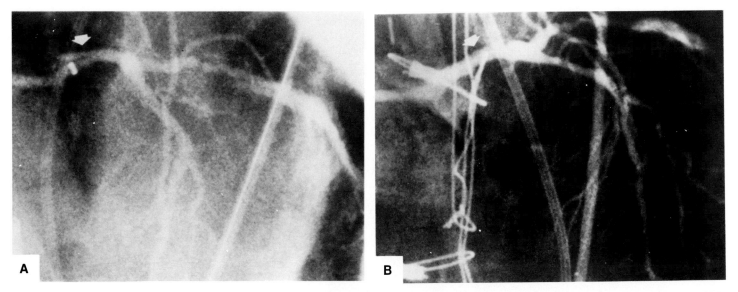

Figure 8-2.4 Guiding catheter-induced dissection of the LMCA is well visualized in an LAO-cranial view (A, arrow). Because the LMCA was protected (patent LAD graft), the dissection flap was successfully tacked down by prolonged balloon inflations as seen in (B, arrow).

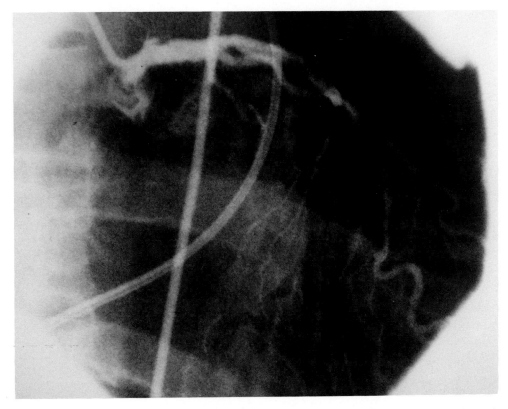

Figure 8-2.5 A proximal LMCA dissection at the distal tip of the guiding catheter is indicated by a dye staining cap on the superior border of the LMCA. Such dissections often occur when the guiding catheter size is slightly smaller than ideal, causing a marked upward pointing of the guiding catheter. A larger curved catheter might have been able to be positioned in a more parallel fashion to the axis of the LMCA. No complications occurred and the patient recovered well.

8-3 GUIDE WIRE FRACTURE

An infrequent complication of intracoronary intervention is guide wire fracture. This occurs most commonly when the distal wire tip becomes entrapped in a chronic total occlusion or in a small distal branch. Usually, it is associated with extensive guide wire rotation or forward push, although occasionally the wire may unexpectedly become entrapped or migrate distally. Early recognition of wire entrapment is most important and can be detected when the tip fails to move as attempts are made to rotate or withdraw the wire. Removal of the broken wire, using a balloon over-the-wire technique, is described in Figures 8-3.1 and 8-3.2.

Guide Wire Fracture

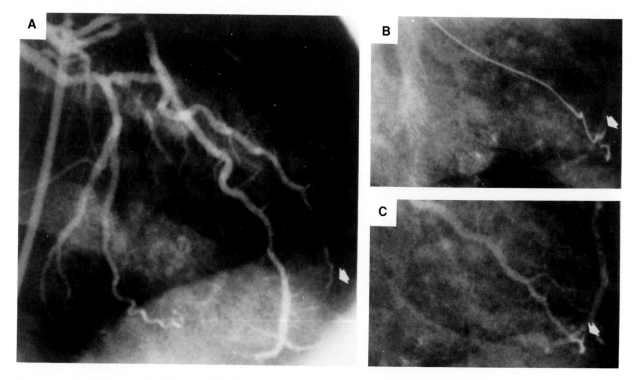

Figure 8-3.1 In this RAO (15°) view (A), there is a significant lesion in the ostium of a large LCX marg branch with marked distal vessel tapering (arrow). The guide wire was inadvertently advanced too far into this very small distal branch and became entrapped. (B) indicates fracture of the distal tip of the guide wire (closed arrow). Once the remainder of the guide wire was removed, a small distal remnant remained in the vessel (C). Noting the course and the complexity of the coronary artery is important in order to avoid wedging of the wire tip and to allow careful removal of the trapped wire. Removal of the entrapped guide wire should be attempted by advancing a balloon catheter as close as possible to the broken segment and by removing both wire and balloon catheter simultaneously. It is important to recognize wire fracture so that appropriate attempts can be made to avoid leaving fragments behind.

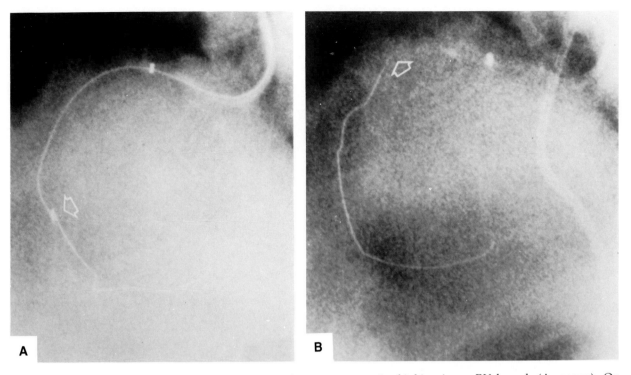

Figure 8-3.2 This LAO-cranial view of the RCA shows extreme wire kinking in an RV branch (A, arrow). On attempting to withdraw the guide wire, fracture was noted. Because of total occlusion, the wire could not be removed completely. (B) demonstrates the proximal end of the wire (arrow) with no extension into the aorta. Contrast injection demonstrated persistent total proximal RCA occlusion (nonacute). No further attempt to remove the wire was performed as there was no adverse effect on flow and the wire did not extend into the aorta.

8-4 VESSEL PERFORATION

Native coronary artery or vein graft perforation is uncommon. While coronary rupture with tamponade is always a concern, most ruptures are self-contained, particularly when angioplasty is performed after previous coronary artery bypass surgery. Major factors leading to coronary perforation include (1) disproportionate ratio of balloon or device and native artery size, (2) excimer laser angioplasty, and (3) sometimes, guide wire perforation. Dissection associated with ELCA is not uncommon; however, major perforation is rare (Chapter 7-2). Perforation due to guide wire manipulation, although infrequent, is most likely to occur during attempts to cross a chronic total occlusion. Angiographic recognition of coronary perforation is important because of the associated risks of tamponade or vessel closure from a compressing hematoma. Figures 8-4.1 and 8-4.2 describe examples of coronary rupture and their management.

Angioplasty-Induced Coronary Perforation

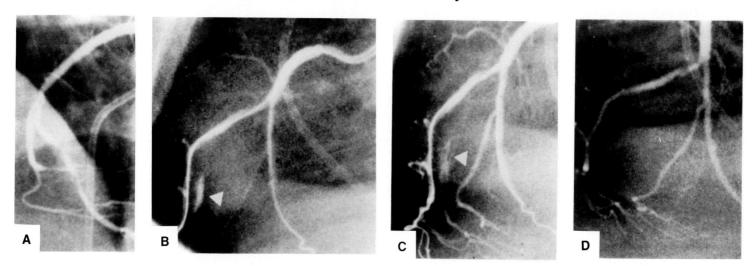

Figure 8-4.1   A large RV marg, terminating at cardiac apex with multiple lesions, is seen in an LAO-cranial view (A). PTCA of the mid-lesion was complicated by development of a pinhole balloon leak causing local vessel rupture with extravascular contrast staining (B, arrow). The visceral location of the stain was best visualized in the lateral projection (C). Although the patient experienced chest discomfort, no ischemic ECG changes were documented. (C) shows partial resolution of the stain 15 minutes later, which entirely resolved in 30 minutes. An echocardiogram demonstrated normal RV wall motion and no pericardial effusion. (D) is a similar lateral view at 1-month follow-up showing no late adverse angiographic abnormalities.

Coronary Perforation With Pericardial Tamponade

Figure 8-4.2   In this shallow RAO view (A), there is a critical lesion in the mid-portion of the LAD. After PTCA and adjunctive DCA, repeat angiography (B) demonstrates an aneurysm at the site of the DCA (open arrow) and evidence of dye staining in the pericardial space (closed arrow), requiring urgent pericardiocentesis. The RAO-cranial view (C) shows sealing of the perforation after prolonged balloon inflation, using a perfusion balloon catheter.

9

Special Considerations

9-1 LEFT VENTRICULAR FUNCTION

LV function is an important consideration in coronary intervention. First, overall extent of global function relates to the risk of both bypass surgery and interventional therapy. Assessment of segmental function may be very important in identifying the sequence of interventional revascularization (ie, the vessel supplying the more ischemic or depressed LV segments usually requires initial treatment). Furthermore, it is important to note that ventricular dysfunction is not always permanent. Many depressed zones, particularly in the distribution of a high-grade lesion or in the setting of an unstable ischemic syndrome are potentially reversible. Thus, recognition of the characteristic thrombotic lesion morphology in the distribution of an abnormal segment in conjunction with the clinical history of unstable ischemia may suggest potential reversibility of the depressed segment. Figure 9-1.1 demonstrates recovery following revascularization.

Recovery of Left Ventricular Function

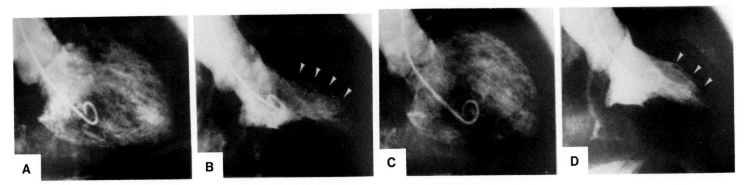

Figure 9-1.1   This is an RAO view (A and B) of end diastolic and end systolic frames that demonstrate an area of significant hypokinesia in the anterolateral wall of the left ventricle in a patient with recent unstable angina and a significant LAD stenosis. Similar RAO views (C and D), 2 months after successful PTCA of the LAD, demonstrated recovery of systolic function in the anterolateral wall of the left ventricle (arrows).

9-2 PERIPHERAL ANGIOGRAPHY

Peripheral angiography of the distal aorta and ilio-femoral vessels is important to the interventionalist in assessing the possibility of vascular complications, particularly when considering the use of devices that require larger guiding catheters (eg, DCA, RA, stent placement) or intra-aortic balloon counterpulsation. In addition, vascular access in many of the more elderly patients may be complicated by extreme tortu-osity or significant atherosclerotic disease, which can increase the risk of vascular complications. In the presence of severe peripheral vascular disease, additional vascular obstruction from coronary catheter insertion may produce local limb ischemia. In such patients with limited vascular access, peripheral angioplasty or stent placement may be necessary prior to coronary intervention. Examples of peripheral vascular disease, which highlight the importance of preintervention assessment and management, are included in Figures 9-2.1 to 9-2.8.

Distal Aorto-Iliac Atherosclerotic Disease

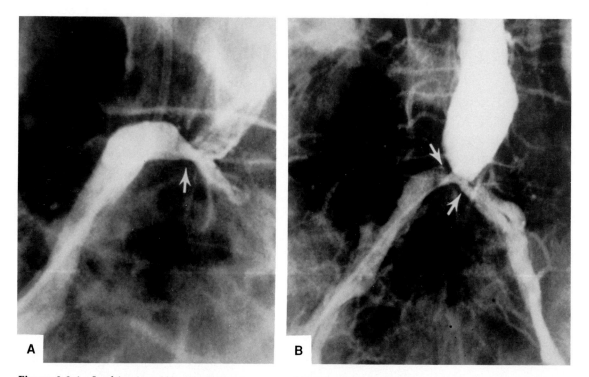

Figure 9-2.1 In this view (A), arterial access was achieved using the Seldinger technique. An 0.038 in J curve wire was advanced to the iliac bifurcation but could not be advanced into the distal aorta. A right Judkins diagnostic catheter was introduced over-the-wire and selective contrast injection was performed, revealing a high-grade ostial iliac stenosis (arrow). A PTCA guide wire was then introduced through the diagnostic catheter and steered across the iliac lesion using angiographic guidance with test contrast injections. The diagnostic catheter was then carefully advanced into the distal aorta and the PTCA guide wire was exchanged for a standard 0.038 in wire. In this view (B), an abdominal aortogram performed later in the study revealed high-grade bilateral iliac stenoses (arrows).

Vascular Access in Patients with Severe Iliofemoral Disease

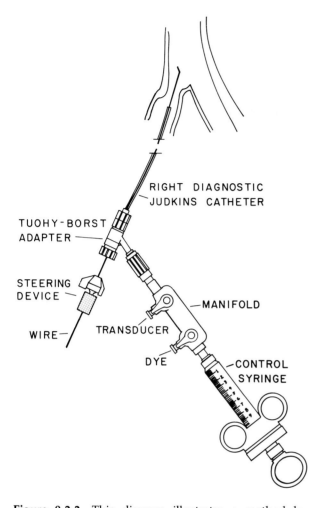

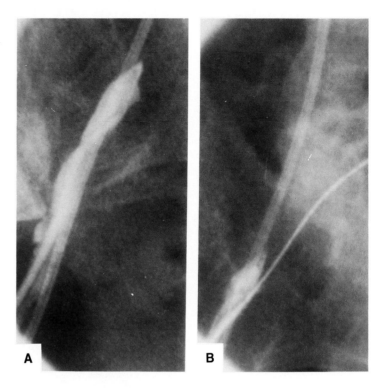

Figure 9-2.2 This diagram illustrates a method by which tortuous or diseased iliofemoral vessels can be traversed using a steerable PTCA guide wire with a tuohy-borst Y occluding device in association with a diagnostic right Judkins catheter. This technique allows for contrast testing and pressure monitoring during guide wire passage and catheter advancement beyond the obstruction. Using fluoroscopic guidance, care must be taken not to kink the PTCA guide wire while advancing the diagnostic catheter. Furthermore, once the PTCA guide wire is freely advanced into the upper abdominal aorta, it can be reinforced by an SOS wire before advancing the diagnostic catheter. Alternatively, a TAD wire (0.035 in wire with a tapered 0.018 in flexible steerable tip) can be used to provide better catheter support for advancement, particularly in tortuous vessels, although the ability to test inject through the catheter is reduced. (Reprinted from Evelyne Goudreau and George Vetrovec. A technique to access severely diseased arteries. *Catheterization and Cardiovascular Diagnosis* 26:53–54, 1992. Copyright © 1992 by *Catheterization and Cardiovascular Diagnosis*. Reprinted by permission of Wiley-Liss, a division of John Wiley and Sons, Inc.)

Figure 9-2.3 Illustrated here is an injection into an apparent blind pouch in the right iliac artery, although there was systemic arterial pressure consistent with antegrade flow (A). However, a standard 0.038 in wire would not advance beyond this point. (B) illustrates dye testing, showing the blind pouch with the PTCA guide wire being passed slightly rightward and advancing well into the abdominal aorta. The right Judkins catheter was then easily advanced into the central aorta. (Reprinted from Evelyne Goudreau and George Vetrovec. A technique to access severely diseased arteries. *Catheterization and Cardiovascular Diagnosis* 26:53–54, 1992. Copyright © 1992 by *Catheterization and Cardiovascular Diagnosis*. Reprinted by permission of Wiley-Liss, a division of John Wiley and Sons, Inc.)

Vascular Access in Patients with Severe Iliofemoral Disease

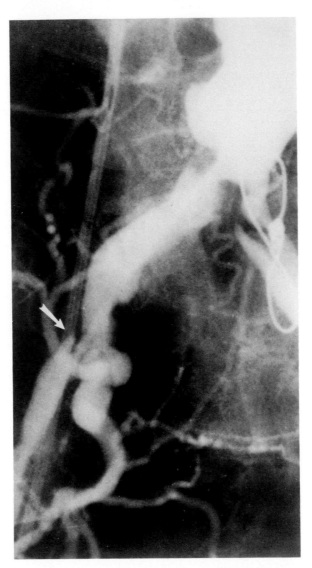

Figure 9-2.4 A later abdominal aortogram of the same patient identifies the blind pouch (arrow) that made routine wire passage difficult. Use of the described technique made vascular access safe and reduced the risk for vascular complications. The following Figure 9-2.5 shows the same patient. (Reprinted from Evelyne Goudreau and George Vetrovec. A technique to access severely diseased arteries. *Catheterization and Cardiovascular Diagnosis* 26:53–54, 1992. Copyright © 1992 by *Catheterization and Cardiovascular Diagnosis*. Reprinted by permission of Wiley-Liss, a division of John Wiley and Sons, Inc.)

Diffuse Aorto-Iliac Atherosclerotic Disease

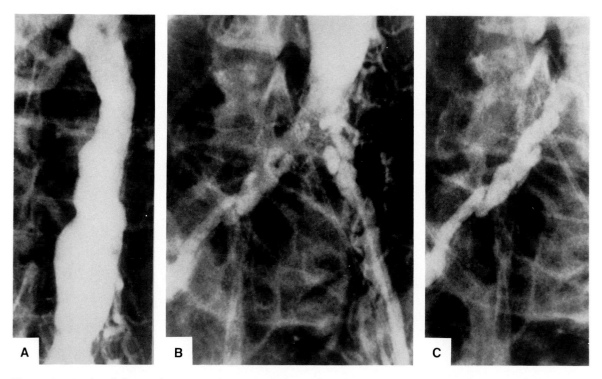

Figure 9-2.5 An abdominal aortogram reveals diffuse atherosclerotic disease of the distal aorta (A). A later phase abdominal aortogram (B) reveals severe bilateral iliac lesions representing contraindications to potential intra-aortic balloon pump insertion. (C) is a more selective injection of the right iliac artery, which shows very diffuse and severe iliac disease. Such screening at the time of diagnostic angiography is useful in ultimately planning the type of interventional device that may be utilized. It is also useful to determine the arterial approach for further interventional procedures and the safety of using intra-aortic balloon pump counterpulsation should the patient become hemodynamically unstable.

Abdominal Aortic Aneurysm

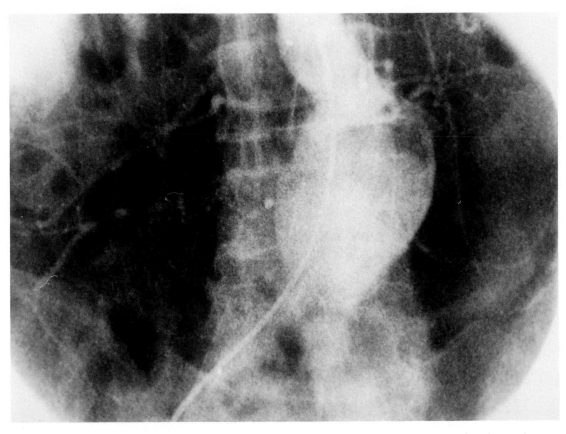

Figure 9-2.6   A screening abdominal aortogram reveals a large, previously unsuspected, infrarenal aortic aneurysm. While sizing of the aneurysm is limited because of potential intra-aneurysm thrombus, recognition of asymptomatic aneurysms can be important in considering the use of large guiding catheters or intra-aortic balloon pump counterpulsation.

Femoral Artery Pseudoaneurysm

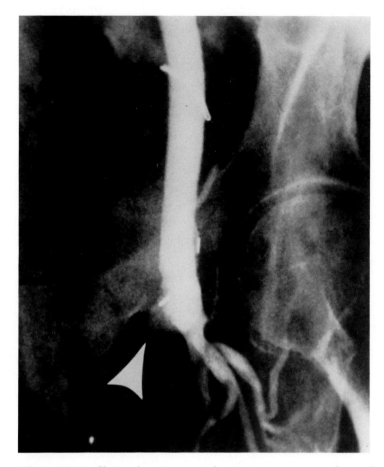

Figure 9-2.7 Shown here is a pseudoaneurysm at an aortofemoral graft distal insertion site (arrow). The pseudoaneurysm was palpable and may have resulted from prior arterial femoral access at this site. If not enlarging, painful, or causing emboli or neuropathy, repair may not be necessary. However, if possible, one should avoid subsequent arterial access in this region.

Femoral Arteriovenous Fistula

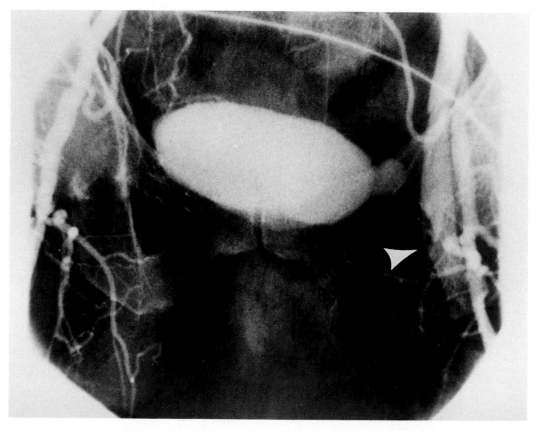

Figure 9-2.8 This late phase of an abdominal aortogram reveals venous filling adjacent to the mildly but diffusely irregular left femoral artery. The exact point of AV fistula formation could not be clearly identified. Small fistulas may close spontaneously if they are recent, while large fistulas require surgical repair.

9-3 RENAL ANGIOGRAPHY AND ANGIOPLASTY

Renal artery stenosis is an increasingly recognized phenomenon that contributes to hypertension, particularly in the elderly population. Screening abdominal angiogram performed at the same time as coronary angiography, is simple, not time-consuming, and very low-risk. These studies can potentially provide useful information regarding the possibility of significant proximal renal artery stenosis in patients with renal insufficiency or poorly controlled hypertension. In addition, relative renal size can be estimated from the renal shadow seen following contrast administration. When necessary, selective renal angiography can be performed utilizing either the RCA catheter or an IMA diagnostic catheter. The latter may be advantageous because of the often downward direction of the renal arteries, which may be more easily cannulated by the sharper curve of the IMA catheter. Examples of renal artery disease and successful angioplasty are shown in Figures 9-3.1 to 9-3.5.

Bilateral Renal Artery Stenosis

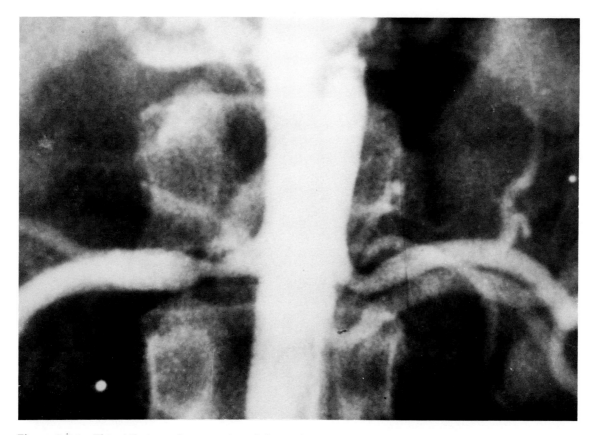

Figure 9-3.1 This AP view of a screening abdominal aortogram performed at the same time of coronary angiography shows a significant lesion in both renal arteries. Note that, at times, slight LAO angulation may provide improved assessment of both renal arteries. Nearly 20% of patients with hypertension who undergo screening abdominal aortograms will have significant renal artery stenosis. The incidence increases in patients with renal insufficiency.

Assessing Renal Size

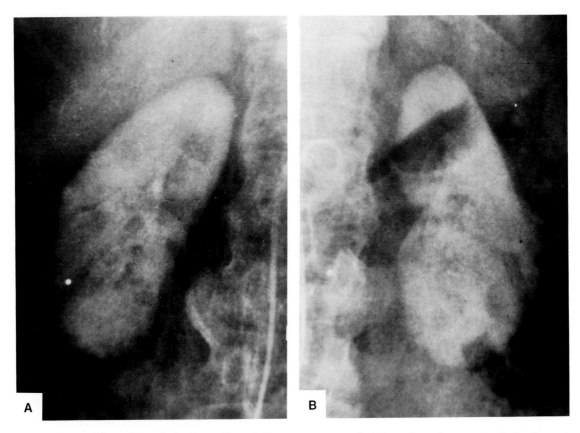

Figure 9-3.2 Bilateral renal shadows (A and B), postcontrast administration, show normal-sized renal structure, despite significant bilateral renal artery stenosis in the same patient as in the above illustration. Note the detail is quite sufficient to assess overall kidney size.

Bilateral Renal Angioplasty

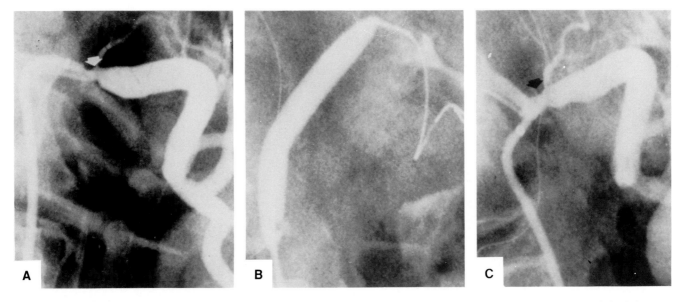

Figure 9-3.3 Selective injection through a guiding catheter (A) demonstrates a significant lesion at the ostium of the left renal artery. (B) illustrates balloon inflation across the lesion. Follow-up angiography (C) shows a significant improvement in the luminal narrowing at the ostium of the left renal artery.

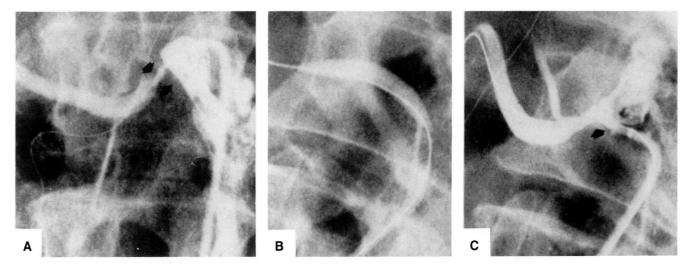

Figure 9-3.4   A severe tubular proximal right renal artery stenosis (arrows) is shown in (A). Note reflux of contrast around the guiding catheter into the distal aorta and late filling of the otherwise relatively smooth right renal artery. Balloon inflation is illustrated in (B). Follow-up angiography seen in (C) shows mild residual narrowing.

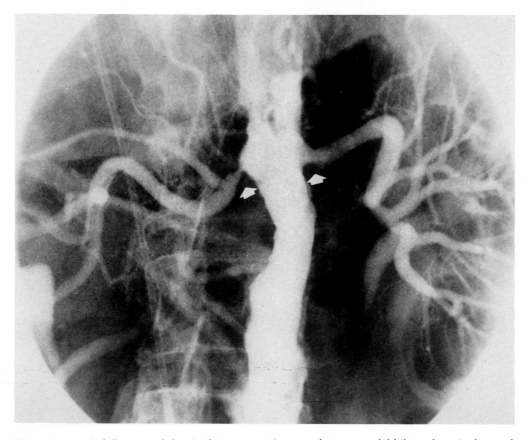

Figure 9-3.5   A follow-up abdominal aortogram 2 years after successful bilateral angioplasty of the same patient, revealed significant restenosis of the right renal artery but no significant residual narrowing of the left renal artery. Renal function remains within normal limits and the blood pressure remains controlled without medication. Restenosis of ostial, atherosclerotic renal artery disease is common following balloon angioplasty.

9-4 SUBCLAVIAN ANGIOGRAPHY

As noted in the section on IMA assessment (Chapter 4-2), the subclavian artery has become important to the interventionalist because of frequent use of the IMA as a coronary graft conduit. Thus, lesions involving the subclavian artery can have an impact on coronary perfusion. To this extent, careful and appropriate angiography and angioplasty of the subclavian artery are important to achieve improvements in coronary flow for selected patients. Examples of subclavian angiography and angioplasty are included in Figures 9-4.1 to 9-4.3.

Proximal Subclavian Artery Stenosis

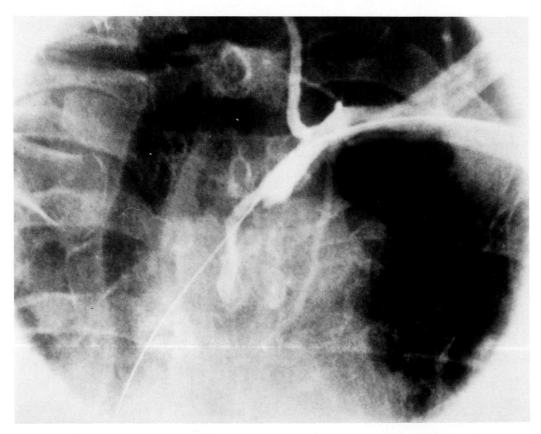

Figure 9-4.1 Shown here, in a shallow LAO view, is a proximal, eccentric, tubular, left subclavian artery stenosis from the left arm approach. A guide wire is seen advanced into the central aorta and there is faint filling of the LIMA anastomozed to the LAD. Optimal views to visualize subclavian stenosis often require testing several angulations to best identify the extent and severity of the lesion.

Subclavian Angioplasty

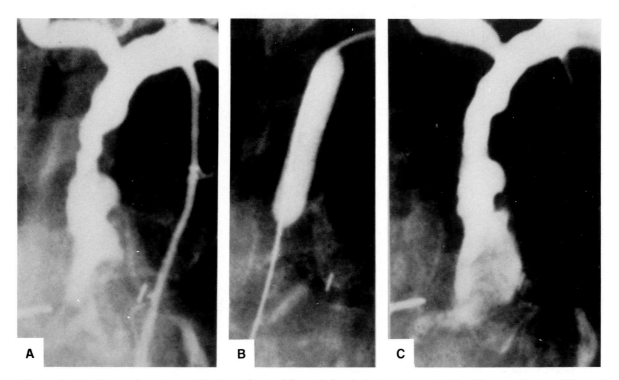

Figure 9-4.2   Shown here is an AP view of a significant left subclavian stenosis (A) with nonselective filling of the LIMA. A similar AP view (B) illustrates balloon inflation across the stenosis and (C) illustrates follow-up angiography, revealing improvement in the stenosis with resolution of the translesional gradient.

Special Views for a Tortuous Subclavian Artery

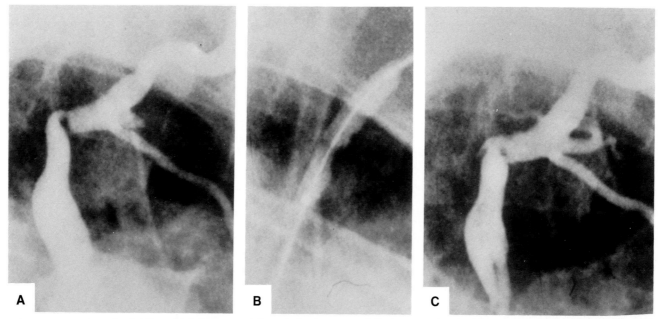

Figure 9-4.3   Standard AP and LAO views of the subclavian artery failed to reveal a significant stenosis despite a 40 mm Hg gradient in a patient with anterior ischemia post-LIMA graft to the LAD. However, in a steep RAO-caudal view, a very eccentric, focal subclavian stenosis is clearly visualized (A). Similar views illustrate balloon inflation (B) and the follow-up result (C). Following balloon inflation there was no residual gradient. The patient became asymptomatic.

10

Summary

With the advent of interventional techniques, coronary angiography quickly became routine; however, this text has attempted to reemphasize the importance of high-quality angiography particularly in the interventional era. Unfortunately, excellence in angiography does not just happen. Angiographers must have a basic awareness of coronary anatomy as well as specific angiographic views and techniques that maximize coronary visualization. Most important, the angiographer-interventionalist must have a commitment to excellence; that is, the willingness to spend additional time to utilize the most appropriate catheter for optimal coronary opacification, to take the single additional view to be certain a vessel branch point is well opacified and to verify that the final PTCA result is really adequate in more than one view. Consequences of this additional effort include improved patient and device selection, interventional outcomes, and better recognition of potential or existing complications.

To this end, it is hoped that this text will help all interventionalists, both beginners and experienced operators, to achieve optimal angiography and interventional outcomes.

Glossary of Abbreviations

AP	Anteroposterior		LMCA	Left main coronary artery
AV	Arteriovenous		LV	Left ventricular
CABG	Coronary artery bypass grafting		Marg	Marginal branch
DCA	Directional coronary atherectomy		PDA	Posterior descending artery
Diag	Diagonal		PLB	Posterior lateral branch
ELCA	Excimer laser coronary angioplasty		PTCA	Percutaneous transluminal coronary angioplasty
Fr	French			
IMA	Internal mammary artery		RA	Rotational atherectomy
LAD	Left anterior descending		RAO	Right anterior oblique
LAO	Left anterior oblique		RCA	Right coronary artery
LCA	Left coronary artery		RIMA	Right internal mammary artery
LCX	Left circumflex		RV	Right ventricular
LIMA	Left internal mammary artery		UK	Urokinase
LM	Left main			

Index